To: George Anne

From: Peggy

NOTHING'S CHANGED

DIARY OF A MASTECTOMY

NOTHING'S CHANGED

DIARY OF
A MASTECTOMY

Dorothy Abbott

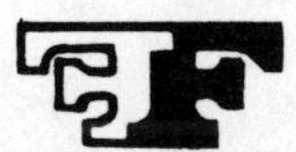

Frederick Fell Publishers, Inc.
New York, New York

For information address:
Frederick Fell Publishers, Inc.
386 Park Avenue South
New York, New York 10016

Library of Congress Catalog Card Number: 81-65746
International Standard Book Number: 0-8119-0423-7

Printed and Bound in Canada

1 2 3 4 5 6 7 8 9 0

For my Bosom Buddies,
with admiration
For my doctors,
with gratitude

Altered names conceal the identities of persons
mentioned in this diary.

NOTHING'S CHANGED

DIARY OF A MASTECTOMY

It's not so bad!

This is what I want to stress: *It's not so bad.*

We women are conditioned to panic at threat of mastectomy. Old wives' tales warn of repelled lovers, dissolved marriages, diminished sex drives, crippled arms, mental breakdowns, even suicide.

But mastectomy need not be a shattering ordeal. Many women claim their post-operative years are their happiest and most fruitful. After facing the reality of cancer, a woman finds it easy to separate her truly important goals from mere busy work.

Cancer is fearsome, of course. Friends who rallied to my hospital bedside asked questions that reflected their own inner panic. *If it happened to you, Dorothy, it could happen to me.*

Which is shockingly true. When I began this diary in November, 1978, one woman in thirteen was destined to develop breast cancer during her lifetime. The 1981 statistics released by the American Cancer Society alter this estimate to one in eleven.

One in eleven!

So there are a mighty lot of people with breast cancer in their futures.

Yes: people. Men, too, get breast cancer, and in a particularly virulent form, their cases making up about one per cent of the total.

There will be 111,000 new cases of breast cancer in the United States in 1981, a two thousand increase over the 1980 forecast. Breast cancer deaths in 1981 will number 37,100, up

1,100 from the previous year. For the vast majority of new cases, a mastectomy will be advised.

How does a mastectomy affect a woman, her husband, and her children? How badly does it hurt, physically and emotionally?

"It's not so bad," I told my friends who visited me at the hospital.

They weren't convinced.

To prove my point, I began this chronicle of my own experience. It is my personal story. Some women may breeze through mastectomy more easily than I. Others may suffer more and heal more slowly, God love them.

JULY 1978–NOVEMBER 1979

JULY 1978

Early July

Four Months Before Surgery

I never have been diligent about examining my breasts for lumps.

Why not? I wonder in retrospect, for I don't have a head-in-the-sand personality; I prefer to face up to trouble and battle it.

But mine is not a cancer-prone family. We die heart-first. Besides, there is something narcissistic about a woman's poking and stroking herself. . . .

Excuses! Excuses!

To my shame, it is pure luck—or the guidance of God—that puts my left fingers to my right breast when my right arm is stretched high overhead. This is the only body position in which the lump can be felt.

It seems as if the hardened stub of a cigarette is lodged there, in the fat at the bottom of the breast, in what medically is termed "the lower outer quadrant."

There is a similar but less pronounced oddity in the left breast, which alleviates my suspicion. I am confident that cancer doesn't exist in matched pairs. *When is a lump not a lump?*

My annual physical examination is scheduled for November. "I'll mention this to Dr. Clarkly then," I promise myself.

But every day I poke at the spot, wondering. . . .

I am an obedient patient, reporting annually, earning accolades at my continued bloom. At this point, I am fifty-two, playing tennis, walking vigorously for my health, taking Disco lessons—feeling better than ever before in my life.

I am too healthy for cancer.

Later In July

My conflict rages. *Shall I go to the doctor now, or shall I wait until November?*

I like my doctor; I don't want him to peg me as a wolf-crier.

Yet I have been brain-washed by the American Cancer Society. Their Seven Warning Signals are etched in my memory. Number four reads, "Thickening or lump in breast or elsewhere."

But is mine a lump? I consult with friends who have undergone biopsies.

"There would be no doubt in your mind," they assure me. "It is like a marble, and you can move it around."

I have no marble. Instead I have a cigarette stub, or a slim segment of Tootsie Roll. It is like a muscle, maybe, or a rope. It doesn't wiggle. It is anchored snugly.

Therefore it is nothing, I console myself.

I keep the lump secret from Louis, my husband, and the lump in its turn conceals itself from him.

Every day I poke, tweak, and test. . . . Indecision shadows me.

I credit God with being a nag. About ten days after discovery I phone my doctor's office and learn Law One about breast bumps: *No delay*. My appointment is set for this afternoon.

Friday, July 14

With his nurse as chaperone, Dr. Clarkly does his finger-dance across my breasts. I lie on his examination table and apologize, "This isn't anything. I'm embarrassed at being here."

"Don't ever be hesitant," he says. "I want you to come in when something shows up."

He is a good man. He is a kind man.

"But there are *sick* people in your waiting room," I protest, feeling guilty at wasting his time. Then I wince as he fingers the peculiar rope in my breast.

"You have poked that spot till it is sore," he scolds. "Now don't poke at it any more! Just check it once a month."

After the examination, I dress and meet him in his office. Sun is beating through a glass door onto his jungle of potted plants.

My chair is solid against the floor. His swivels. Somehow that puts him at an advantage.

Our eyes meet.

He says, "This doesn't have the look of cancer."

"No," I agree. Any other statement from him would have astonished me.

He continues. "Perhaps I am being over-cautious, but because of your age I think we should go ahead and get X rays."

My age. That stinker. He is every bit as old as I am.

The significance of needing X rays doesn't panic me. In twenty-five years, Dr. Clarkly never has lied to me. He says no cancer; he means no cancer. What's more, he knows that he needn't shield me. Having shared several episodes of pneumonia with me, he knows I can shoulder trouble without freaking out.

While I listen, he phones the local radiologists, then apologizes to me. "Since this is Friday afternoon, it will be Monday before we can get you in."

"Fine." Already I am accustomed to Law One regarding breast bumps. The medics are in a hurry, but I am not.

I carry Dr. Clarkly's order for a mammogram away from his air-conditioned office into the blast-furnace heat of a southwestern summer. How I love this heat!

I feel marvelous. I have been a good girl: I have taken my lump to my doctor. He is being a good boy: he is playing it safe. We both know nothing will come of this.

My lump is a false alarm.

Monday, July 17

Three patients are in the radiologists' waiting room when I arrive so I settle down with *The Wall Street Journal. The Wall Street Journal?* Never before have I seen it in a medical bailiwick. I suppose cancer victims, undergoing treatment here, check the health of their investments. Poor guys. The suspicion that I, myself, might be a cancer victim is totally absent.

No doubt my lack of fear is a protective device, an indulgent gift from my brain or from God, Who always has been generous with me.

A woman in a no-nonsense uniform jacket appears from the mysterious back rooms.

"Mrs. Abbott," she says crisply.

The three patients ahead of me shift in their chairs. No other Mrs. Abbott stands.

"Mrs. Abbott," the woman repeats, impatiently.

With a shrug of apology to the others, I follow her, mumbling, "Law One."

The dressing rooms are like facilities at the beach and equally charming. I am fed into a square cubbyhole with its floor area hogged by a molded plastic chair, ugly and cold. Even at 115 pounds I am crowded.

The hooks for hanging clothes are sharp, slim talons. I eschew their danger and drape my outfit over the chair as I don a frayed gown.

How fault-finding and crabby I am! Am I afraid, after all?

I try to interest myself in the supplied magazine, a gossipy rag on the opposite end of the spectrum from *The Wall Street Journal,* but it fails to divert me.

Mercifully soon, I am fetched and taken to an X-ray room, where I allow myself one quick and nervous belly-laugh. Prominent on the wall is a sign, *"We have the hardest beds and the worst drinks in town."*

Fortunately, a mammogram doesn't require the swallowing of a nasty beverage. What it requires is a seated patient positioned so her breast rests in a certain way on that advertised "hard bed."

That hard and *cold* bed!

The technician pays much attention to the height of the stool, swiveling it up, swiveling it down, then up again. Likewise, she adjusts the X-ray "bed" up and down.

My left elbow is placed, just so, on the cold surface. I am instructed to lean forward and brace my weight, just so, so that my breast flops onto the table, just so.

The problem is, I don't have floppy breasts. Back in dormitory days I was classified "cupcake" when it was fashionable to be "cantaloupe" or "watermelon." Alas.

The camera pushes its cold nose against my flesh.

But things still aren't right. The technician nudges my breast hither and thither like a reluctant glob of clay. She shapes my breast to her specifications with wedges of foam rubber.

I am in shock. My modesty is coming unglued.

Can this be me, submitting without protest?

She works diligently but futilely.

I say, "I'm sorry to be such trouble. I'm sorry I'm not bigger." I've been sorry about that since age 12.

"We have trouble with the big ones, too," she admits, unhappily.

With that, our dialogue dies.

The "positioning" continues.

I force myself to think about the sands of Puerto Vallarta until I remember its traditional name: Beach of the Dead. So I switch channels in my brain to concentrate on the Alps, on San Francisco, on anything, anything except this indignity.

A sign of progress comes when the technician plunks a small metal marker beside my breast. It is inscribed "R" to indicate the right breast.

To guard against amputating the wrong boob, I joke to myself, refusing to take this scene personally. Amputations are for the unlucky and the ill, and I am neither.

Demanding that I quit breathing, the technician ducks into her protected cage and grinds out her picture.

"You can breathe now," she allows generously.

Then she repeats the entire routine to X-ray my left breast.

"But my lump is on the right side," I protest.

To no avail.

I wait in the X-ray room with its corny, ominous sign until the films are developed.

I flunk my screen test.

The technician returns with reinforcements. Now two women in no-nonsense jackets swivel the stool, raise and lower the "bed," nudge flesh with foam rubber, guide the giant camera. There is some dialogue about getting the nipple in profile.

In profile! Like a face in a cameo.

Again I flunk, and we launch a third round of pictures.

X rays make me nervous. Aren't they, in themselves, rumored to be cancer causing?

Three times proves a charm. With the news that my pictures finally are adequate, I am ushered to an examining room. One of the trio of radiologist partners, Dr. Pelt, arrives to poke my breasts. His finger-dance is different from Dr. Clarkly's.

He announces, "This is normal breast tissue."

Of course it is! I have known it all along. I don't even feel relief because I have been so confident.

I pay my $60 bill and leave. Fast. The mammogram experience has not been a highlight of my day.

But it does make an amusing story to tell Louis. "I had a little lump I didn't tell you about, but all is well." I relate the technicians' difficulties.

Neither Louis nor I voice the word *cancer*.

NOVEMBER 1978

Monday, November 6

Ten Days Before Surgery

Dr. Clarkly's jungle of plants threatens to take over his office. How they have grown in just four months!

Cheerfully I greet him. "Here I am again, cluttering up your office with my robust good health. Every year I feel better and better."

"I wish I could say the same." He sighs.

Pity etches into me. He is an old-style, dedicated physician who doesn't spare himself. How tired he looks! The white in his dark hair no longer is a hint. It is a fact.

I'm not exaggerating: I feel great. My allergies are under control. The fatigue that plagued me as a younger woman has subsided. Perhaps I am demanding less of myself. Certainly my responsibilities are diminished now that my children are grown and away.

I threaten, "Don't you dare ferret out any fresh problems!"

Like a good girl, I answer his routine questions. Like a good boy, he makes jottings in my Manila folder. We both know I'm healthy as a horse.

Since this is the day of my annual physical, I know I can't avoid a pelvic examination, that old favorite of women everywhere.

I go to his examining room to undress.

"Doctor wants to check your breasts, too," his nurse informs me.

My breasts! Absurd as it sounds, I have forgotten the anxiety caused by that stub of cigarette anchored so firmly to the base of my right breast. Oh, now I check it monthly. This laudable habit is the pay-off from my July scare.

The examination progresses nicely, and I figure I am free and clear for yet another year. Then comes the exploration of my breasts.

Dr. Clarkly spends a lot of time at it.

I reflect, this isn't too hideous an experience. My lifelong modesty is ebbing.

En route to the door and escape, Dr. Clarkly says, "Dorothy, I believe that lump has grown."

"It's normal breast tissue," I argue.

"To be on the safe side," he soothes, "I'll order another mammogram."

Oh, for pity sakes!

"Not this week," I stipulate. "This week I'm baby-sitting my grandson."

Thursday, November 9

Seven Days Before Surgery

Louis announces that my priorities are wrong; I can hire a sitter for our grandson. On the edge of being angry with me, he subscribes to Law One without knowing that it exists.

At his insistance I phone for the "earliest possible appointment." Today is the day.

There is more pushing and shoving of my bosom. More nudging with foam rubber wedges. More dialogue about getting the nipple in profile. More photographic repeats when "takes" fail.

During the whole ordeal, I dwell on the much-publicized, doctor-denied theory that X ray itself causes cancer.

On duty in the examining room today is a younger radiologist, whose technique when he examines my breasts is different from the others.

He retreats across the room before he speaks. "We see nothing on the mammogram."

Of course you don't! So what am I doing here besides leaving behind another $60?

"But for your age, your breasts are very dense," he says.

"Like my head." Truly, I am annoyed at myself for being here, when I could be at home playing Snoopy's Doghouse with my grandson.

Instead, I am playing this young doctor's game. I ask, "What does that mean—*dense?*"

"It means the X ray isn't getting through the tissue. We don't pick up the lump with X ray—but, of course, we feel it."

We. I have visions of medical multitudes lining up to prod my lump, to squint at my secretive X rays.

He pronounces, "A woman your age. . . ."

My adrenalin flows. What does my age have to do with it? I feel great, really great! I'm not sick, that's for sure, and I'm not going to let any youthful doctor talk me into being sick.

Besides, fifty-two is The Prime of Life.

He is saying that my lump doesn't have the look of cancer, but to set everybody's mind at ease, I ought to have a biopsy.

A biopsy! What nonsense. A hospital stay is involved, and an anesthetic, and all that operating room rigamaroll. Besides, my friends with their wiggly marblelike lumps emerge from biopsies free and clear, so why bother in the first place?

I plunge into battle. "I have read that mammograms pick up tiny cancers too small to be felt."

"This is true," he agrees.

"Then how could it miss a lump as big as mine—if mine were cancer?"

It is a question that I am to ask over and over during the next months until, finally, my dense brain grasps the fact that dense tissue does, indeed, block X ray.

I ask questions which the young radiologist patiently answers. I argue.

He stands firm in his recommendation for a biopsy.

"But we have reservations!" I wail. "For a week from Saturday. We're going to go sit on the beach in Mexico."

Dammit, I AM going to sit on that beach in Mexico, I promise myself.

"Then have the biopsy when you get home," he suggests.

When I get home. So there's no urgency! Without urgency, there is no threat. . . .

So, all right, I'll play the doctors' game. But first I'll go sit on the beach.

Friday, November 10

Six Days Before Surgery

MORNING: In this city, Thursday is doctors' afternoon off. It is Friday before the radiologist's report reaches Dr. Clarkly.

He phones me.

"Dorothy," he begins, and by the sound of his voice, I know I'm in trouble. He concurs with the radiologist. I need to see a surgeon.

"The mammogram is negative," I argue.

Dr. Clarkly says, "A woman your age. . . ."

A woman your age. Medically, I grant, this phrase is not a putdown. Yet, with its every repetition, hot blood speeds to my ears, deafening me. I love being my age; I feel great physically and emotionally.

Dr. Clarkly is telling me that from a biopsy will come a "frozen section" that will rule out the possibility of cancer.

"The mammogram is negative," I repeat, clinging to a fragment of hope. I don't like hospitals.

We discuss my dense breasts. How can a woman who hasn't skipped a menstrual period in twenty years have an old woman's breasts? At my prodding, Dr. Clarkly describes the denseness as something akin to scar tissue.

Scar tissue. I know darn well why scars form. The body has marvelous healing powers, and scars mend something that is wrong.

What could be more wrong than cancer?

AFTERNOON: In keeping with Law One, a surgeon agrees to see me this very day. He is new to our city, and I know nothing about him.

His waiting room is harvest-decorated in anticipation of Thanksgiving. I love Thanksgiving. Twice before, Louis and I have observed the holiday in Mexico. This year, too, we will be there. Basking, baking, tanning in the sun.

Oh, I am anxious to get going! I will appreciate the vacation all the more because of this small scare.

In an examining room, I put on a paper jacket.

"Fine," the nurse says, "except you have it on backwards."

So, unlike fanny-exposing hospital gowns, this jacket opens in the front. Where the breast is.

"Of course," I agree. "How stupid of me."

Once the door shuts behind her, I am off the examining table and prowling the room, suffering no nervous moments because I am too busy enjoying the place. On the walls are antique medical and pharmaceutical signs, battered and faded —and funny. Also, there is an old fashioned printers' tray mounted on the wall, its compartments which once separated type now creating frames for miniature, medical-related doodads. In the cubbyholes are tin patent medicine boxes, an ancient and lethal-appearing hypodermic syringe, a cough drop package I remember from my childhood, and gadgetry still older, dating back to the turn of the century.

Hey, how old is this surgeon, anyhow? Will he dodder into this examining room dressed in high-top button shoes and a Celluloid collar? Well, what matter? For my own sake, I couldn't care less about the steadiness of his hand in the operating room; after all, I'm here on a false alarm.

So I savor his display of amusing miniatures as fast as I can, because this is my one and only chance. I won't be coming back, at least not until I'm much older, at least not until I have a *problem.*

The door opens, and Dr. DeHaven, the surgeon, enters.

An emotional fist punches my belly. *He is 15 years old.* He is tall, lanky, and blond, the date every girl covets for the high school prom.

I can't avoid comparisons: My former surgeon also was my much-loved friend, a mature man, and he has died.

Of cancer.

The youthful surgeon examines my breasts, and I grant he knows his stuff. He is the fourth medic to prod at me since July. By now I am a qualified judge of technique.

"Well, I guess you'll have to show me this lump," he concedes.

I catch my breath. *He can't find it! It's gone!*

He waits.

"I have to lift my arm," I offer, doing so.

And then, indeed, the lump is there.

He fingers it, squeezes it, jabs it. . . .

"It doesn't have the look of cancer," he judges.

Oh, those beautiful words!

"I know," I agree happily. "Nobody thinks it does." Suddenly I am liking this youthful doctor and deciding not to give him a bad time, unless he mentions, "A woman your age. . . ."

He says, "If I were the first to see this, I would say, wait and watch. But Dr. Clarkly has been waiting and watching. So we will go ahead with the biopsy."

I jump into battle. "The mammogram is negative." Then I introduce the subject of scar tissue.

The term "scar tissue," he assures me, is Dr. Clarkly's effort to explain denseness in layman's language, and the scar tissue in my breasts is not my body's effort to repair itself. So, I have jumped to a conclusion and worried needlessly! How I have worried! So foolishly. I determine to pursue answers to my questions hereafter, until no cobwebs of misunderstanding remain.

An admirable goal.

But for me, it isn't going to work. In the months to come, I will again and again tangle myself in mistaken notions. Repeatedly, I will translate physicians' "layman's terms" into dire prognoses. I will suffer self-inflicted and needless torment.

Dr. DeHaven speaks of my upcoming biopsy, qualifying, "A woman your age. . . ."

Does every doctor in town have a hangup over my age? I interrupt with knives in my tone. "We've got reservations for Mexico. To sit on the beach."

"Well, go ahead," he urges calmly, agreeing with Dr. Clarkly and the young radiologist. "We'll tend to this when you get back."

There! No urgency! Therefore: no cancer.

Reluctantly, I admit, "My husband says I have warped priorities. He says he can't enjoy a vacation with such a doubt hovering. He says that I'm to enter the hospital in robust health—and that's not the way I return home from Mexico."

Dr. DeHaven says nothing.

"But Mexico is worth it!" I insist.

Then I demand, "Give me the figures. How confident are you that this isn't cancer?"

He hates my question and replies reluctantly, "Ninety-five per cent certain."

"Well, that five per cent doesn't scare me," I brag. And it doesn't. I am separate from this, as if we are discussing some stranger.

We have a choice of two procedures, he tells me. One, I can go to the operating room for a biopsy and only a biopsy. Then in two or three days, after all laboratory tests are complete, if cancer is found he and I together can decide how to treat it. Alternatively, I can be kept under light sedation after biopsy, until a frozen section is analyzed. "If it shows cancer, the surgery can proceed," he tells me.

"You mean, chop off the breast." My words are sharp.

"That's not a description I favor."

"But if I select biopsy only," I muse, "and there is cancer, I still lose the breast. That is the treatment you favor, isn't it?"

"From all the statistics, all the evidence. . . . Yes, I feel the best chance to eliminate breast cancer is to remove the breast."

"So the big surgery merely is delayed," I point out.

"If surgery is the route you choose."

We are going in circles.

"Why have anesthesia twice?" My tone is brittle. "If I have cancer, please do the whole job at once." I feel over dramatic and silly, as if I am emoting in a poorly-written melodrama.

I can't tell if he approves of my decision.

He opens my Manila folder. "You are scheduled on Thursday morning."

Scheduled! All that nice-guy encouragement about taking my vacation—while all the time, he has me scheduled!

Thursday is six days away. A truly soothing fact. No urgency: no cancer.

Monday, November 13

Three Days Before Surgery

What rotten timing. Now I have a bladder infection! The urgency to urinate plagues me all night. When I can delay fifteen minutes between trips to the bathroom, it is a victory of mind over matter.

About midnight, Louis escapes to another bedroom, and I don't blame him. At 3 A.M. I remember the sleeping pills on the top shelf, but I refrain. Drugs frighten me.

Tuesday, November 14

Two Days Before Surgery

When my internist's appointments clerk arrives at his office, I am there waiting, a mayonnaise jar of "specimen" in my hand.

Dr. Clarkly is at the hospital, of course; no telling how long I will have to wait.

I get chummy with the technician because I pass her laboratory en route to the bathroom, time and time again.

Slowly Dr. Clarkly's waiting room fills. Because of my supreme seniority, I am first to see him.

He holds my lab report in his hand. "All you have," he informs me, "is a case of nerves. The specimen is negative."

Wednesday, November 15

Day Before Surgery

At the ridiculous hour of 9 A.M., three of us check into the hospital for surgery tomorrow.

"Dr. DeHaven likes his surgery patients in here early," the volunteer at the admittance desk comments.

I mutter beneath my breath.

My co-victims are a man of about sixty and a woman of uncertain age, handicapped by extreme obesity. She is accompanied by an overalls-clad man who walks in pain, and I am accompanied by Louis, who doesn't quite trust me not to abscond to Mexico, although I have pledged good behavior.

For each of us, there is an office where we reveal the identities of our insurance companies and various deep secrets, such as our ages. I sign a permission paper for surgery; I am signing away the ownership control of my right breast.

Back in the lobby, the man patient is gone. An aide comes with a wheelchair and settles the obese woman into it although her husband is more needy of the ride. I wince at his pain as the three of them depart.

I wait.

In time, the same aide returns.

I'm not getting into that invalid's chair! We put my luggage into it and our guide pushes. We trail her. As we bypass the elevator, my hopes rise. Double doors loom ahead.

I recognize the area. "It's the 'Holiday Inn!'" I cry, joyous. This is the new wing, designated "self-help." Each room is a single with private bath. Furnishings are motel-modern except for the high bed.

An aging, brusk nurse lays down the laws of her domain. "Nobody down here eats in bed," she decrees. "You eat right here." She pounds her fist on my desk. "Down here, you take care of yourself. We carry your trays, we make your bed— but that is all."

"Suits me," I say, intending to burden nobody. Just take that defective chunk out of my breast, I think, and let me go about my business.

Softening somewhat, the nurse explains the intercom built into the wall at the head of my bed. She shows me the button that lights the bulb outside my door. Not that I'm to call a nurse with it, apparently.

Then as proudly as if the architectural design had been hers, she leads me down the hall to where the nurses' station jags to the right, a small lobby to the left. What a wondrous place! In addition to furniture and magazines, there is a compact kitchen with a bottomless coffeepot, a spigot that gushes boiling water ("Be careful not to test it with your finger; it always is boiling hot!"), packets of instant soup and instant coffee and instant cocoa and instant whatnot, and a refrigerator stocked with fruit juices, pop, ice cream. . . .

All is for the patients' use, twenty-four hours a day. I am impressed.

Louis goes to work, and I return to my room. A short distance from my window are the fenced yards of private homes. A heavy grayness hangs in the air; this is not the typical brilliant, sky-clear day I have come to expect and crave here in the southwest. Sunshine is my joy. As if in sympathy, the sun will emerge only once in the next ten days, the days of my hospital confinement. There will be much rain. My tennis chums will insist I'm missing nothing during this imprisonment.

But I'm allowed no time to gaze into the future. Admittance wheels are spinning, and a volunteer arrives to escort me to the lab.

"Annette!" I cry.

"Dorothy!"

We have known each other for twenty years.

She asks, "What are you in for?"

"Biopsy."

"Breast?"

"Yeah."

"Both of my breasts are gone." Annette might have been saying, "I had eggs for breakfast."

"I won't need a mastectomy," I assure her. "My lump isn't cancer."

"We'd better get down to the lab," she says.

The older man and the obese woman are waiting for us at the elevator. Annette is shepherding us all.

The elevator arrives. It is deep and wide, to accommodate gurneys—the hospital word for a stretcher on wheels. *Tomorrow I'll be on a gurney in this elevator, heading to surgery. . . .* Goosebumps chill my spine, yet I'm still cocooned by the drug of unreality: *This can't be happening to me.*

In the elevator, the obese lady and I establish rapport; she is friendly and talkative. "I'm in for my gall bladder. I put it off six months, but I can't put it off any longer," she tells me.

"Well, good luck," I say.

"What are you in for?" she persists.

This sounds like prison dialogue. I want to reply, "Arson," or "Kidnapping," but of course I don't. Subdued because the man is listening, I choke out, "Breast."

Heat rushes to my cheeks. When I was growing up, we didn't say *breast.* Come to think of it, we don't say it much nowadays, either. We say *boob.*

The man mumbles the only words I ever will hear from him. "You don't have to hunt far to find somebody who's worse off than you."

He means me! He thinks I'm in jeopardy of my life!

Before I can reassure him, the elevator door wheezes open. Immediately I'm in an atmosphere of love. Three of my close friends are medical technicians here; their children raised, they now are working.

Their warmth is edged in concern, and I recall that Christy has lost both breasts to cancer and Bertha one. So certainly statistics are with me. Cancer can't happen to all of us.

Annette sends me into a cubicle to fill a specimen jar. Christy draws my blood and—surprise!—doesn't hurt me. Somebody nudges me toward the X-ray department.

"I had X rays last week," I protest.

"We need new chest X rays before surgery."

This is so that there are no surprises like TB or pneumonia to be discovered on the operating table, I learn later. So I lose that battle but win the electrocardiogram war since my last is only nine days old. I hope that my insurance company appreciates my efforts on its behalf.

The day spins on. Not a lot happens. Oddly, I am neither bored nor fidgety.

Lunch tastes great.

I nap on the tall, narrow bed, where Annette finds me. She has finished her duty hours and has come to cheer me. Twenty-five hours between admittance and surgery is too long a span to endure, we agree.

"But there are so many tests to run." She sighs.

As we talk, it becomes apparent that I know nothing—absolutely nothing—about mastectomy. In an act of kindness I shall remember forever, Annette reaches beneath her pink volunteer's jacket and extracts a "prosthesis," a weighted plastic breast form. It is warm from her body heat, and it squishes in my fingers. As I tilt it, its weight shifts and its shape changes, like a human breast in motion.

It is not nearly as repulsive as I might have imagined.

"Just don't puncture it," Annette warns.

Apparently the plastic casing is filled with a gel that leaks, given an opening.

I hold Annette's prosthesis, and we are two women together, close and confiding.

"Your nipples are gone?" I dare to ask.

"Everything's gone!" It is natural and artless that she bares her chest, showing amusing but not unattractive little-boy flatness. A slash of horizontal scar on each side is all that remains where once were fleshy breasts.

"The hospital would kill me if they knew that I was doing this," she says.

In no way do I pity Annette. She is on top of this. She does not pity herself.

But I don't—I can't—link her experience with my life. I am to have a biopsy to silence physicians and my husband; I am *not* to have a mastectomy.

No, sir, not me!

After Annette leaves, I prowl the hall restlessly, peeking into rooms, hunting my obese pal and even hunting the taciturn man. They are nowhere to be found. Apparently, they already are settled on the surgery floor.

Twice, Dr. DeHaven comes with his giant penicillin needle, a precaution against infection in a flawed valve of my heart. I am happy to see him despite the needle. We are buddies by now.

Dinner is good.

All food is good, I have noticed, if I don't cook it myself.

Louis arrives to spend the evening. We are companionable together, just like at home. Our television remains blank and silent, just like at home. *Thank goodness I have no roommate!* Hospital roommates are always deaf and adore television.

A solidly-built young man enters my room and sits on the bed. He is wearing boots. His belt is cinched with an ornate silver buckle. He looks exactly as Southwesterners should, but seldom do.

"I'm Dr. Arnheim," he introduces himself. "I'm to be your anesthesiologist."

"You're an important person in that operating room," I tell him.

"You know your stuff!" He goes on to explain, "I'm going to give you a light anesthetic, as light as possible. Both for the biopsy—and in case we need to go farther."

"You won't," I assure him. Then I grumble about missing Mexico.

"My mother is there now," he says.

"You rub salt in my wounds," I complain.

Enough small talk. He eyes me. "What is your mental attitude about this surgery?"

I say, "Good" and Louis says, "Bad," all in the same breath.

"Don't listen to him," I beg. "I'm feeling fine."

He believes me, apparently, because after his departure a nurse posts a sign above my bed. It reads, "No pre-op sedative."

Thursday, November 16

Day of Surgery

MORNING: *Why doesn't Louis arrive?* I open my door to gaze hopefully down the hall, and a booklet plops at my feet. It had been nudged into the door crack.

It is a collection of inspirational quotations with a cover notation from my minister: "Sorry I missed you."

Missed me? I haven't budged from this room. And how I am hungering for a gesture of loving attention, some comforting warmth—yes, some intercession with God on my behalf!

How have I missed my minister? How has he missed me?

Then, from dim recollections of my pneumonia days, I recall that a tight-shut door is a hospital code: doctor in attendance, or treatment being given, or simply "No Admittance." I had shut the door and my pipeline to God.

Well, no matter. This isn't a crucial day in my life. Rather, this biopsy falls in the nuisance category. It is inconvenient, and I am irked.

I sit in my plastic-upholstered easy chair and read spiritual paragraphs although, truly, I don't need them. I'm not frightened.

Louis arrives at last. He isn't late; I have an early start on the day.

There is little to talk about. We are waiting. . . .

Much as I want the dumb ordeal behind me, I'm not yet ready when my door is flung wide to accommodate the scary looking gurney, piloted by an attractive young woman.

"It's only 9 o'clock," I protest. "I'm not scheduled 'til ten." *And Louis just got here. I need more time with him.*

"Doctor is running early." She asks if I'm wearing a dental bridge, bobby pins, rings. . . .

"Just a plain wedding band."

She locks it on my finger with adhesive tape. Then I trade my gown for the clean one that she has brought, and I stuff my hair beneath the shower cap that she gives me.

I ask to walk to the operating room, but this is forbidden. The approved routine, apparently, is to scoot sideways from my bed onto the gurney.

I do as I'm told.

"Nothing to it!" the aide rejoices. "You're not very heavy, are you?"

"115."

"The last patient I moved weighed more than 300 pounds."

I perk up. "That's my friend! Is she O.K.?"

"She came through surgery very well."

The hospital cop-out. Obviously I'll pry no information from this aide.

Oh, well, I'll just see for myself! This afternoon or tomorrow morning, when I'm back on my feet, I'll search the surgery floor for her. I'll tell her my good news, and I'll cheer along her recovery.

In style I roll down the long hall of the "Holiday Inn." Louis walks beside my gurney looking pale and troubled.

I reach my hand to his. My eyes fog over. Oh, I can't die! He needs me.

Of course I don't expect to die. For this brief moment, I am over dramatizing.

The elevator journey takes us smack-dab to the operating room. Immediately, I'm whisked away from Louis. Doors suck shut between us.

Dr. Arnheim, the anesthesiologist, is in the operating room, waiting. Dr. DeHaven, the surgeon, is not.

I ask, concerned, "Did your mother come home with the Aztec Twostep?" I am ready to swap remedies for diarrhea, to practice medicine without a license.

"It's tonight that I go to the airport to pick her up."

"Oh, I thought it was last night," I say, somewhat disappointed.

He is poking a flat thing with prongs at my left upper arm, and I watch with curiosity, knowing our show can't hit the road without the surgeon.

I'm wrong.

Instantly, I'm out-of-it. And I had intended to pray!

HAPPENINGS OF WHICH I AM UNAWARE: Relatives of patients in surgery congregate in a cheerless waiting room, its only redeeming feature a coffee urn. Tension is alive in the air.

It is a particularly difficult chore for some of those waiting, because this is the day of the second annual Great American Smokeout, observed throughout the hospital. "No Smoking" signs are prominently displayed. Many lapels sport "Smoking Stinks" buttons.

From time to time someone tiptoes away, only to return looking guilty and reeking of tobacco.

Louis asks the volunteer in charge, "Is smoking always banned here?"

"Look." She points to the ceiling. It is black.

The volunteer functions efficiently, jotting descriptions—hair in bun, brown suit—so that she can match names to individuals, and send the proper family out to the hall when a surgeon lurks there, ready to report an operation's results.

Those waiting indulge, alternately, in brooding silences and loquaciousness. Famine or feast, with words. It is an Agatha Christie setting—a variety of persons trapped together by chance, with a threatening mood prevailing.

At 9:40, those in the surgical waiting room hear a pathologist being paged. *Right on the button,* Louis thinks, impressed. It is exactly Dr. DeHaven's estimated time for completion of my biopsy.

Over the hump! Louis breathes deeply.

Down in the lab, my dear friend Christy is waiting for the pathologist. She has told him of her concern for me.

He walks past her, carrying my lump in gauze, muttering, "Looks bad."

Christy nearly flakes out. She is more panicked by my cancer than she was about her own. Perhaps this is fair because her cancer, seven years ago, had plunged me into despair. Back then I thought mastectomy was a death sentence.

Christy has a secondary cause for concern. Yesterday, after she typed my blood, she phoned major blood banks in our area only to discover that there isn't a drop of my AB negative available anywhere close. She had delved into her textbooks to double-check that A negative is the best substitute, followed by O negative.

Louis is O negative.

The frozen section shows the pathologist what he has

suspected from the very appearance of my lump—it is cancer.

It is Dr. DeHaven's chore as surgeon to convey the news to Louis.

They meet in the hall outside the surgery waiting room.

"This catches me by surprise," the doctor says. "It is cancer."

Louis admits to feeling, at this point, "Not so good." Also he remembers being unsurprised, having considered my chances all along as 50/50, despite Dr. DeHaven's guess at 95/5, and despite my negative mammogram.

Dr. DeHaven tells Louis, "We will remove the breast now. This is what your wife wants." He adds that my blood is the rare AB negative. He doesn't expect that I will need a transfusion, but if I do another blood type can be substituted.

This information does nothing for Louis's peace of mind.

"It should take me about another hour and a half," Dr. DeHaven estimates.

An hour and a half! Ninety minutes of uncertainty, turmoil, and fear.

Kindnesses occur even at the worst of times. Louis is diverted by a parade of visitors: my internist Dr. Clarkly who registers his surprise, the always-cheerful gynecologist, who is a tennis buddy, Evelyn from the lab, Christy from the lab. . . .

"She will have good days and bad days," Christy warns, speaking from expertise and experience.

In ninety minutes Louis and Dr. DeHaven again meet, and Dr. DeHaven reports, "All is well."

Relief apparently digs a hole in my husband's stomach. Through ears blocked with emotion (or is it hunger?) he hears the doctor say, "She is in the recovery room now, and we'll keep her there about an hour. We'll let you know when we move her to her room."

"Has the cancer spread?" Lou's question is abrupt, demanding.

"I've been wrong once today," the doctor says, "so I'm not going to speculate further. I'm not going to say the axillary lymph nodes are cancer free—but they do look that way. We'll know more in twenty-four hours when the rest of the tests are complete."

With an hour at his disposal, Louis hurries to the hospital cafeteria and devours a giant lunch.

How disloyal! Worry, after all, is supposed to convert prime steak to ashes, ambrosia to dusty feathers. And my husband pigs it up.

In punishment he suffers anxious moments because, after his feast, I am neither in the recovery room nor in my assigned third floor room.

Something has gone awry.

Most optimistic of all possible explanations is that he was told the wrong room number, and he is on his way to the third floor nurses' station to check when a gurney, its protective sides up, is wheeled past him. The patient, gray of skin, is rigged up like an outer-space creature with an i.v. hanging high, dripping into her left arm, and another strange contraption anchored at her right ribs.

Something about that pitiful gray form is familiar, so Louis looks twice, then dares to ask, "Is that Dorothy Abbott?"

Yes, it is I.

Not exactly a beauty, but he is stuck with me.

EARLY AFTERNOON (MY OWN STORY RESUMES): I have no idea what occurs in the recovery room because my first conscious memory is of bossy but compassionate women—a WAC corps of them—insisting that I boost myself from the gurney onto my bed. They harbor a wild, mistaken notion that I can accomplish this under my own power.

"Use your feet," they tell me. "Use your shoulders."

As I float between two worlds, I hear their instructions

and make stabs at obeying, but my brain waves don't reach my muscles. Besides, I'm nailed down by gauze and tape that feels as heavy and stiff as a plaster cast.

I know my breast is gone.

I have no strength to react emotionally. A fact is a fact. So be it.

At last I am in bed and the WAC corps leaves.

I need to hear the truth about my breast pronounced loudly and clearly, to smother a last ash of hope, so I ask Louis my sly question. "Honey, what time is it?"

Aware that my blood pressure is worrisomely low, he postpones discussion until such a time as I'm in better shape. But his subterfuge works not at all. In refusing to tell me the hour, he tells me the whole truth. Only last week we had spoken of brain surgery, remarking that the patient's prompt awakening indicates an inoperable condition—in actuality, a death sentence. For me, a long stay in the operating room is not life-and-death drastic, but it does betoken surgery beyond biopsy. It means *The Big M.*

My breast is gone.

I examine this truth through a fog of left-over drugs, and I accept it calmly, without rebellion. Worse things could happen.

Nurses come; nurses go.

My body is restless. My legs draw up as if from stomach cramps. My knees bend and flex, bend and flex. Pain drills into my right elbow and right wingbone.

I swallow bitter saliva. My head swirls. "I'm going to vomit!" I cry. "Where's that pan?"

A nurse materializes from the far shadows. She nudges the crescent-shaped pan into the angle under my right armpit. I'll have to be a contortionist to use it.

Lou's voice filters from a distance. "She won't vomit. She thinks she is going to, but she never does."

I'm furious at his disloyalty. Can't he see that I'm sick? Can't he understand how lousy I feel?

"I threw up when I had my appendix out," I argue.

"You were seventeen years old," he points out. "That was thirty-five years ago."

His facility at math is not one of my husband's most endearing qualities.

The nurse points out, "Anesthetics were different then." I am surprised that she doesn't preface it with, "A woman your age. . . ."

It will serve them both right when I urpse all over the bedclothes, all over everything. . . .

Of course I don't. Louis is right once again—but only because Dr. Arnheim, the anesthesiologist, is so skilled.

My nausea ebbs away.

I feel pampered—by Louis, by the nurse who pops in regularly, by the aide who takes my blood pressure every fifteen minutes. A new i.v. replaces the old, hanging high above the bed, trailing its nourishment into my left arm. Bloody juices ooze from my body through plastic umbilical cords, collect in a Hemovac, are emptied and measured.

My chest doesn't hurt!

What hurts—plenty—is a lemon-seed-sized spot in my elbow, the too-familiar pinch of tendonitis. Tennis elbow.

I lash out at the next nurse who appears. "Why does my elbow hurt so much?" I wail. "Why does my wingbone hurt?"

"Because of the way your body was strapped onto the operating table," she explains briskly, without tenderness.

I am upset. At this moment, the most important priority in my life is to play tennis. I give no thought to the cancer that might have spread—might require horrendous treatment— might indeed kill me. Only tennis matters.

My knees continue to bend and flex; I can't lie still. I study my new room, a cell compared with last night's lodging. Another cell is adjacent. The two share a common entry hall, shower, and toilet.

I tell Louis, "The radiologists are wrong. They don't have the hardest beds in town. This hospital does."

He fails to wisecrack back. He hardly knows what to say to me. He is as uncomfortable as I am, in a different way.

His shock is more severe than mine.

An aide arrives with her blood-pressure sleeve and paraphernalia, and I appeal to her. "The nurse down at the 'Holiday Inn' said it's not necessary to endure pain. She said I should ask for a hypo when I hurt."

"I'll go see," the aide promises.

A nurse arrives to tell me, "It is too soon."

Louis says, "Wait a bit. You have to wait a bit."

The nurse says, "You have had major surgery and you're supposed to hurt."

She disappears, leaving her words *major surgery* to crumble Louis's fragile wall.

He gathers his resources and tells me my breast is gone.

"I know it," I say, wishing I could ease his pain. I remind him, "You're a leg man."

"That's right," he agrees.

He escapes to the hall for a while.

LATE AFTERNOON: Now that no buffers remain between me and the truth, I settle down. I can wait it out. I feel gray inside and out.

The reason my skin is grayish is because my blood pressure is low. Apparently this indicates continued shock.

My most frequent visitor is the aide with her blood pressure paraphernalia. At her umpteenth check she announces, "Well! It's starting to come up." She is not a candidate for Phi Beta Kappa.

The nurse who denied me a hypo arrives with ice chips for my hot, dry mouth. Nectar—drink of the Gods.

I am uncomfortable, but never, never do I experience the excruciating, mind-wracking pain of a toothache, earache, or menstrual cramps.

At last, I am granted my first hypo. Its effect is fast. It

softens the mattress, soothes my wingbone, calms my elbow. My knees stop jackknifing.

Now that I am comfortable, clouds of time drift softly away. I feel floaty and content.

But I am alert! An expert no less qualified than Dr. DeHaven remarks that, at this stage, I am more clear than most of his surgery patients. He stands at the foot of my bed, and I hear each word distinctly. He says, "I was very surprised. The lump was cancer."

"I know."

I am impressed that he uses the word *cancer*. Never, never will he speak of a "malignancy." A spade is a spade. Cancer is cancer. *Malignancy* is a cop-out word.

He says, "I have removed your breast."

"I know," I repeat.

Why is that tremble in my voice? I'm brave! I'm in control! Admittedly I'm smug about being brave and in control.

"In about twenty-four hours, we will have the final lab report," he promises.

My alertness, fortunately, doesn't extend beyond the current moment, so I am spared the twenty-four hours of nervous waiting endured by Louis. The report will indicate whether the cancer has invaded my underarm lymph glands—the axillary—the usual route for the spread of breast cancer.

With involvement of the lymph, I will undergo cobalt (X ray) therapy and/or chemotherapy. With no lymph involvement, I will go my merry way, on the tennis court and elsewhere.

Dr. DeHaven warns, "Now don't raise your arm above your head."

As if I would! As if I *could!* I feel like Mack-the-Knife's victim, encased in cement.

He adds, "I'm ordering a liquid dinner for you."

Hot ziggety! I'm making progress.

When the doctor leaves, I confide in Louis. "I do think he's older than fifteen. Twenty-five, maybe?"

Dinner is a bomb, and only partly because I can't sit up. The mushroom soup is so rich it gags me. The shimmering, sparkling cubes of orange jello hold no allure.

Still flat on my back, I spend a few lifetimes on the bedpan. The skill of functioning in this fashion always has eluded me, and eludes me still. The nurse returns with terrible tubes and remarks at the quantity of urine I surrender.

After she leaves, I have to go to the bathroom more desperately than before. I decide that I'll never, never again take a toilet, or my ability to use it, for granted.

Louis has endured about as much "hospitalization" as he can. "I'll go home now, and let you sleep," he decides, kissing me on the cheek.

On the cheek! I demand and achieve better.

I sleep marvelously the whole night through.

Friday, November 17

Day After Surgery

DAWN: I awaken.

I'm alive!

The gauzes and tapes of my bandage imprison me, but there is no pain. Actually I feel great!

Except today is no different from any other bright new day. Familiar urgencies signal me. I punch the button to call the nurse.

She arrives, prompt and smiling. And why not? Her shift nearly is ended. In an hour she can go home.

I grin back at her. "Will you help me get to the bathroom?"

Her smile fades. "You're just one day post-op. How about using a bedpan?"

"I tried that last night. No way. . . !"

"It's only 6 A.M.," she protests.

"It's *today*, isn't it? Dr. DeHaven said I can get up today."

I read her face: *Why do I always get these crazies on my shift?*

"I'll see," she promises.

Perhaps she carries my challenge to higher authority. Anyhow, when she returns she is accompanied by a white-clad buddy.

It takes both of them, plus my total concentration, plus 110 per cent of my strength to extract me from the high bed. We aren't dealing merely with my abused, rubbery body. Accompanying me is the i.v. pouch attached by tubes to my left arm and the Hemovac attached by tubes at my right ribs.

For eighteen hours the i.v. solution has oozed into me. No wonder some of it wants out!

On my way back to bed, I catch a glimpse of my suitemate. She is fantastically frail and might easily be a hundred years old. Her relatives are assembled from far-away places to take turns staying with her around the clock.

All signs indicate that this is her last family reunion.

MORNING: Breakfast is my first real meal, and I devour orange juice, oatmeal, and buttered toast with no concern for calories. I eat propped up in bed, Queen of the Castle. I am proud of myself.

At eight, Louis arrives.

"Don't you have to go to work?" I ask.

"Work can wait," he says.

He loves me! Even now, with a splendid part of me chopped off, he loves me.

At ten o'clock Suzanne, our older daughter, tiptoes into my room.

"You're here!" I exclaim. "How come?"

"How could I teach—when this happened to you?"

Tears blur my sight. *She loves me, too.*

Everybody loves me. I love everybody.

Louis says, "Since Suzanne is here to keep you company, I'll go on to the office."

"Wait! Help me to the bathroom first."

He shows no enthusiasm.

"It takes two to get me there," I confide.

So with Suzanne on my left, holding the i.v. high, and Louis on my right, handling the Hemovac gingerly, we shuffle to the bathroom.

"I'm not dizzy," I brag.

"Since when?" Suzanne challenges.

AFTERNOON: Every cancer patient needs a time for introspection, and this is mine.

There has been much—too much—material in the press about the emotional effects of mastectomy. Statistics are kept on post-mastectomy suicides, divorces, alcoholism, drug dependency, unhappiness. . . .

These don't touch me. These *won't* touch me. Here I am in a hospital bed, as free from fear as I am free from pain. My future remains rosy, as it always has been.

Rosy, very definitely.

The root of my security is in the character of my husband. He is strong emotionally, as level-headed as God creates any man. He won't be repelled when he views my new body—my body with the subtraction. Of course, he will be sad—I want him to be sad. That right breast has been part of our private, closed-door lives for thirty years.

Fortunately he is an avowed Leg Man. I shall keep reminding him of this.

I shall keep reminding myself.

Here in the hospital I am feeling no panicky regrets for what-might-have-been in my life. The abrupt time-is-running-out terror that must strike some cancer victims is not touching me, because I encountered my personal crossroads earlier, on my fiftieth birthday. It was then that I quit paving toward some obscure "future" and began living totally in the present: saying "No" to perfectly reasonable demands on my time and talents, and concentrating on what delights and satisfies me.

This selfishness has brought me contentment without hurting anybody. Editors may miss me, but they buy other people's stories; organizations flourish without my leadership; the health department has not yet condemned my back closet.

My breast cancer emerged at the usual age, in mid-years. Its appearance any earlier might have horrified and angered me. As it is, my emotions are cushioned by a half century of experiences.

I am hopeful rather than fearful—but, *Dear God, I don't want to die!*

LATE AFTERNOON: It is a glorious day; the i.v. is taken away. Now it seems easier to cope with the Hemovac as it dangles from my right ribs.

Louis and Suzanne are with me in the late afternoon when Dr. DeHaven arrives. Standing at the foot of my bed, he wastes no time in preliminaries.

"I have a good report." His grin is wide. "We took out twenty-nine lymph nodes, and they all tested negative."

Louis and Suzanne react physically, as if they have been holding their breaths since yesterday morning.

"This means," explains Dr. DeHaven, "that you won't need cobalt or chemotherapy treatment."

"Oh," I squawk, for I have not programmed myself ahead that far. My immediate concern has been the pain of my tennis elbow; my long-range concern has been whether I can play again, come spring.

He tells me to walk the hospital halls, to swing my arm from the shoulder.

"Ow," I predict, accurately.

When he leaves, my daughter says, "I'm impressed with your doctor."

"He's too old for you," I kid. "He's pushing thirty."

NIGHT: My roommate's family turns off her TV when *Tora Tora Tora* ends. They say goodbye, leaving a representative to settle in for the night.

My own visitors leave.

I am very tired; I am ready to sleep.

But the hospital is rampant with noises. Across the hall a woman with a piercing, nasal voice screams, "No, Mother, you're not at home. You're in the hospital. I'll stay with you tonight, Mother. Tomorrow Emma Lou will stay with you. . . ."

I expect a nurse to hush that shrill monologue, but it continues, the same message, over and over. My roommate, bless her, gives no trouble. But beyond my other wall, somebody is gasping grotesquely for breath and wheezing—or perhaps merely snoring? It sounds alarmingly like noises I make when I have pneumonia, and my lungs ache in sympathy.

I have no pain, but I am uncomfortable. My skin grows east and the adhesive tape pulls west. I can't find a comfortable position. I wonder if I ever, ever will be able to sleep on my stomach again.

Too, I wonder if my obese friend and the taciturn man are asleep, down on the surgery floor. Is it more quiet down there? The hospital is running full, and my room is on the medical floor, which I love because the glass-enclosed nursery is within my walking range. I'm a pushover for babies.

Sleep eludes me. After much time passes, I push the button for the nurse.

"I can't fall asleep," I complain to her. "It's too noisy."

"You can ask for a hypo."

"I don't want a hypo."

"You're only one day past surgery."

"Just shut the door," I beg.

"It's against the rules," she says. But as she leaves, the stopper that props the door ajar fails. The door wheezes shut.

Suddenly it is darker and a little more quiet. I doze. Then there are screams in the hall, and sobs that penetrate my shut door. Voices wail in a Greek chorus. When the nurse makes her hourly round, I pry for information. Unsuccessfully.

The next afternoon I read in the local paper that a young woman with teen-aged children died during the night at this hospital. Cause of death is not listed, but memorial contributions are to go to the American Cancer Society.

I am grateful my children are grown.

Saturday, November 18

Two Days After Surgery

MORNING: I have a playful admirer. He grips my lost bosom. He tweaks my lost nipple.

I name him Agrippa.

He is a surprise to me; nobody warned me that I would experience phantom pain.

Agrippa attacks swiftly, with no minor twinges of warning beforehand. As rapidly as he pinches, he retreats. At times he strikes every few minutes; at other times, he is mysteriously absent for hours (leading his Roman legions to another battlefield?).

In our weeks together, I grow vaguely fond of Agrippa.

I never can grow fond of the raw discomfort in some interior structure whenever I swallow liquids that are either icy cold or piping hot. How sore it is deep inside there! It will be a month before this annoyance ebbs.

Traffic into my room is heavy. Nurses show a bizarre interest in the blood-colored contents of my Hemovac, that flat flask attached beneath my right ribs by transparent plastic tubes to collect the juices that ooze from me. The nurses empty it on a regular schedule, measure, record their findings. . . . Dr. DeHaven calls the contraption a purse, I call it a flying saucer, and nurses with scant imagination call it a Hemovac.

Each day the oozings will be less red until, on the sixth day, they are yellowish and meager, and the Hemovac at last is removed.

But this is just the second day after surgery, and I have a long way to go.

My day's first visitor is my internist, Dr. Clarkly, on whom I unload the miseries of my sleepless night. I tell him a hospital is no fit place for sick people. Because he is kind, above all, he responds to this hoary observation with good-natured agreement. At least he admits that mine is a universally-held opinion.

In his wake comes Dr. DeHaven, merrily announcing, "This morning I'm going to change your bandage." He peels the west-tugging tape from my east-growing skin, discards the bandage, and pauses.

A very long pause.

What is he waiting for? What am I supposed to do?

Am I supposed to LOOK?

I want to look. How I want to look! But my curiosity is tempered by caution. Thus far, I have been a "Class-A Heroine," a "Courageous Fighter in the Face of Adversity." Dare I risk my reputation now? I mistrust the depth of my own courage.

So I continue to stare at the ceiling.

The new bandage is small and comfortable, and the new adhesive tape gives me no trouble whatsoever.

His bandaging finished, Dr. DeHaven says, "I'm going to send you back downstairs."

"To the 'Holiday Inn?'" I can't believe my good fortune. "How wonderful! Thank you!"

He is at my door when I call out, "I don't understand why

I'm not hurting. Isn't a mastectomy considered major surgery?"

He turns, surprise on his face. Obviously he hasn't fielded this question before. At thirty-five, or whatever, he hasn't yet encountered everything.

He says, "Yes, it's considered major surgery, and be glad you're not hurting." He escapes out my door.

I am warned that my move downstairs won't be immediate. Hospitals have check-out times just like hotels.

Lunch is starchy, starchy. On my tray is the menu from which my diet was selected. Oh, how good the vegetables and salads sound! I wonder when I'll be allowed to pick my own food? While I wonder, I gobble every starchy calorie.

Then I am ready for my therapeutic walk down the hall to the nursery. I am excited; I adore babies. I press the button of my electric bed until I am sitting tall. Then with Louis and Suzanne's help, I inch into position until my legs dangle over the edge of the bed. Then I stand—Eureka!

None of this is automatic. I must concentrate hard in order to move. It seems a terrible burden to transport the Hemovac safely along with me.

By chance I own a new and classy bathrobe, red flannel with an appliquéd white cat. Won't I be a bright and cheery fashion plate as I stroll the hospital hall!

Unfortunately this robe zips only part way down the front, and its shoulders are narrow. My helpers puddle it on the floor, and I step into it. With Suzanne on my left and Louis on my right, they tug the red flannel. Uncertainly, I thrust my arms toward the armholes.

Something brushes against my right arm—fabric, perhaps, or Louis's fingertips. The pain is so sudden and so intense that I scream. I scream and scream, like the youngsters screamed last night when they lost their mother.

As suddenly as it started, the pain quits. I am left exhausted. Shock waves chill my flesh. I sag against the bed and weep.

Am I sobbing in grief for my lost breast? I think not. Truly I believe I am surviving mastectomy without tears. No, it is not the breast I mourn but rather the sharp and shocking pain.

It becomes obvious that my best bathrobe, and my second-best, are cut too skimpily across the shoulders for me at this time. Henceforth I am forced to parade the hospital halls in an elderly blue bathrobe, faded and frayed.

AFTERNOON: Suzanne and Louis are at lunch when two aides come to move me downstairs.

"I won't need the wheelchair," I boast. "I'm walking real well."

"Well, you're supposed to ride." For one so young, the aide has an iron jaw.

The second aide loads my suitcase, flowers, and tub of hospital supplies onto a wheeled cart. We look like John Steinbeck's Okies on their way to California.

Our journey covers an impressive distance, and I am thankful to be riding, and that my big mouth hasn't forced me to test my endurance.

My ego is at an all-time high when Louis and Suzanne find me. No question about my progress! I wouldn't be here in the "Holiday Inn" if I weren't healing marvelously, body and soul.

I hold court, pleased with myself. No invalid behavior for me!

When my company leaves, I ask the Hemovac-measuring nurse, "Who will help me get to the bathroom?"

She answers crisply. "Down here, you go to the bathroom by yourself."

What a challenge this presents! Upstairs I have learned to run the electric bed to its most upright position, to wriggle myself across the mattress until my legs dangle, to inch forward until my feet touch the floor.

This technique has no parallel in the "Holiday Inn." Here

the mattresses' ups and downs are maneuvered strictly by manpower—a grinding of the fold-away crank at the foot of each high bed.

Such cranking holds no allure to a right-handed woman two days past right-breasted mastectomy. I am destined to lie however I am abandoned until my next able-bodied visitor arrives.

If only such waiting were possible! But, no. By habit I drink great quantities of liquids, a foolish trait in one handicapped by a bladder the size of a pea. I cannot count on stray visitors to help me out of bed. I must strive to be a big, brave girl and navigate to the bathroom by myself.

The first objective, when I am lying flat or semi-flat, is to hoist myself upright. Of course I can't brace myself on my elbows; my right arm is a clumsy, dead weight that won't abide the pressure of a canary's feather. What's more, my tendonitis screams.

The incision in my chest keeps me from rolling left, from boosting myself with my left arm. There remain the metal railings that convert my bed to a crib, but to tug on them creates a crescendo of pain.

So nothing will work except brutal, physical jerking to an upright position, a procedure with a heavy failure ratio. Jerking brings a pain that is excruciating, just short of intolerable. But unlike menstrual cramps and toothaches and earaches, it fades the instant I am upright.

I complain to nobody. I won't risk being sent back upstairs to the noise and commotion. I am fiercely possessive of this, my very own room.

Besides, once I am sitting upright, my problems are minimal. My slippers I kick aside. Barefoot I step out cautiously but unafraid, and not an iota dizzy.

I do favor my right arm, cradling it in my left arm although Dr. DeHaven wants me to swing it from the shoulder. He is a direct descendent of the Marquis de Sade.

Sunday, November 19

Three Days After Surgery

MORNING: I wake at six, anxious to make my small journey. As I jerk upright, roots seem to rip from my chest.

I squawk in terror. What I have done is forgotten the darn Hemovac. It is trapped in the bedclothes, anchored so that it doesn't follow along with its tubes as I move. I'm sure the contraption is uprooted from my body.

I've undone the whole surgery, I acknowledge. Horrified, trembling, I ring for the nurse. Surely I'm allowed one panic call, even in the self-help unit.

The nurse remains calm as she examines the adhesive tape that conceals the juncture where the tubes enter my body.

"It's O.K.," she judges. "Just be careful hereafter."

Hereafter, I pin the Hemovac to my nightgown, twenty-four hours a day.

LATER: Perhaps it is my fright at the Hemovac accident that turns me melancholy. My concern shifts from my tennis elbow to cancer. *I had cancer. It might recur.* My body chemistry that invited malignancy once might host it again.

Cancer might kill me and God knows, there are kinder ways to die.

Well, I have no desire to die, kindly or otherwise. I'm having too great a time in this world. I want to stick around.

I didn't live those law-school years in a trailer without plumbing so Louis's second wife can wear mink. I'm resenting her hanging different drapes at my windows, hanging different paintings on my walls. Mostly I'm resenting her life with him, because as a husband he is nearly flawless, and already I am jealous of her.

Also I resent that she'll be younger and prettier than I, possibly wittier, possibly sexier.

Don't misunderstand me; I want him to be happy.

I want him to be happy *with me.* I don't think it is the least bit corny to walk into the sunset years hand-in-hand.

Monday, November 20

Four Days After Surgery

MORNING: Peppy and cheerful and feeling great, I am nibbling breakfast when Louis arrives for a brief morning visit en route to his office.

He is cutting my ham when a nurse enters. Glowering, she says, "Sir, I know your heart is in the right spot, but you're not doing her any favors by helping her."

"So I'll quit," he promises.

From this point, there are thorns in my roses. I am forced to use my right arm.

Louis leaves, and I am struggling to take a sponge bath when Jane, my hospital neighbor, wanders in.

"You can't do that yourself," she notices, quite astutely. "Let me help you." When I hesitate, she adds, "I'm a nurse."

"But you've had surgery, too," I protest.

"Just gall bladder. I'd be home now if I didn't have tiny children who want me to pick them up."

So she washes my back and my legs, insisting that she loves to nurse, insisting that she loves to help people.

I recognize her as one in a million. Oh, I have fine nursing care from compassionate women—but Jane is a person apart. We launch a discussion of religion—she is devout, of course. Minutes later I meet her minister.

I horn in. I ask him to pray for me, too.

NOON: Dr. DeHaven arrives to remove my bandages, to expose my chest.

My flat chest.

With the big scar.

I am more curious than fearful because I have viewed Annette's little-boy chest and judged it more amusing than shocking.

But will I be amused when it's my own body that's flat? I'm level-headed, I think, but sometimes my emotions play tricks.

Steady, I urge myself.

The bandage goes.

Bravely, I crane my neck to view my chest.

"I like it!" I tell the startled doctor.

The incision is seven and one-half inches long, an angry red slash from my armpit diagonally to the base of my onetime breast, and an inch short of the midpoint of my body. Most puffy and tender is the bottom inch and a half, the area that tugs most, the area of anguish when I swallow hot or icy liquids.

The slash of incision is a scarlet monorail crossed by ten railroad ties—stitches belligerently black.

"Well, for heaven sakes, it slants," I remark, puzzled. Annette's scars are horizontal.

Dr. DeHaven explains, "It slants because of the location of the growths. I worked from the sites of the biopsies."

"Growths?" I echo, emphasizing the plural. "Biopsies?"

Not only had he biopsied my cigarette stub in the lower outer quadrant, but he discovered and biopsied a lump in the upper inner quadrant. The upper one tested benign.

At the upper end of my incision is swelling and a peculiar flap of flesh, the flesh that stretched flat when my arm was strapped overhead during surgery.

"You can buy a prosthesis that fits around that," the surgeon promises. "It will give a more natural look."

Later when I am learning again to reach and stretch, I will appreciate the flap of flesh because it extends like elastic. Too, it may be the reason I still can wear sleeveless dresses.

Dr. DeHaven warns that exercise, although essential to my recovery, may cause fluid to collect beneath the arm. In case such a swelling occurs, he will aspirate it—remove the fluid—with a needle, by suction. The prospect is less than attractive.

When the doctor leaves, I stand in the privacy of my bathroom and examine my one-breasted chest in the mirror. I feel a brotherhood with the cyclops, who had one eye, and the unicorn, who had only one horn.

AFTERNOON: One of my visitors is Franny, a long-time friend who underwent mastectomy in the days of the disfiguring radical operation. And no wonder the radical earned such a black name! Franny's incision remained open and oozing a full year after surgery, and she suffered much pain in her upper left leg where a big patch of skin was removed for a chest graft. Today, much of her leg remains unpigmented.

"I don't wear shorts," she remarks wryly.

Between visitors, I am daring enough to venture to the hospital's gift shop, off the lobby. Who should be lingering in the lobby but Glen and Harriet, my neighbors? They are checking Glen in. He is to have a growth on his larynx removed.

He tells me, "If it is cancer, there is a ninety-seven per cent cure rate in this area."

Cancer! Oh, dear God, not two cancers on the same block in the same week!

Glen is assigned overnight to the "Holiday Inn," and I go to welcome him and Harriet to turf I consider my own.

He expresses sympathy at my loss.

"It isn't so bad," I insist. "Fortunately Louis is a Leg Man."

"Then it's a good thing they didn't saw off your leg," he declares immediately.

Oh, how it hurts to laugh!

EVENING: In the lobby of the "Holiday Inn," I introduce Louis and Jane. "She gave me my bath this morning," I boom appreciatively.

Will I never learn to keep my big mouth shut?

Louis and I travel to the third floor to pay our respects to the babies. I am wearing my ratty blue bathrobe with the Hemovac safety-pinned at my hip.

Up on third, ambulatory patients are strolling the hall. Plodding toward us, gingerly and reluctantly, is the taciturn man who had checked into the hospital when I did, who had shared my elevator ride to the laboratory that day before surgery.

"Nice to see you!" I gush. "How are you feeling?"

He snarls.

This completes our dialogue.

Louis says, "He's not happy, is he?"

"He's hurting." I force myself to swing my arm so I, too, hurt.

Because every baby in the nursery is sound asleep, I suggest a pilgrimage to the gift shop. There we meet Isolde who, pregnant, is about to teach a class in natural childbirth.

She eyes my Hemovac. "What happened to you, Dorothy?"

"I had cancer, and I lost a boob."

When Isolde moves on, Louis remarks, "We don't think alike."

"Since when?" I question, laughing.

"You said you lost a boob. I would say you lost a breast."

So I don't say *boob* in front of him again, but I think it, because even this small, limp joke alleviates the solemnity of my surgery.

Tuesday, November 21

Five Days After Surgery

MORNING: I have a drug hangover. Despite my better judgment, I swallowed a sleeping pill last night. It is my choice whether to accept a pain pill, a sleeping pill, or nothing.

I prefer to opt for nothing, but I haven't been sleeping well here in the hospital. No doubt it is because I am a stomach sleeper, restricted by the nature of my surgery to laying on my back or left side.

Brain-fogged and sluggish, I am no match for the day-shift nurse who marches into my room at 7 A.M., announcing, "You were overheard!"

I was overheard. My stomach knots. From the nurse's behavior, it is obvious I have said and/or done something contemptible, despicable, deplorable, scandalous. . . .

But what?

Her words sting, like shotgun pellets. "You are down here in the self-help unit for the purpose of taking care of yourself. This is for your own welfare. You are not to enlist the aid of other patients." She gasps for breath, then booms at me, "You are to take your own bath!"

"Oh, that," I say, immensely relieved. From the force of her judgmental anger, I had been braced for the revelation of a much greater sin.

This all seems silly and vague, anyhow. The drug veils my world.

Apparently I am not contrite enough. She stands tall as she announces, "I am going to report this infraction to Dr. DeHaven and to Jane's doctor. You will hear from them."

There are pains in my chest. My stitches are ripping. I haven't been chastised like this in years.

"Keep Jane out of it, please," I beg. "It isn't her fault." *And*

*she is employed at this hospital. I can't bring trouble down
on her.*

The nurse makes it clear that it is her duty to squeal on
both of us—we sinned and we must atone.

She leaves.

My foggy brain can't sort out this puzzlement. If I were
upstairs, a nurse would be bathing me. Some doctors use the
"Holiday Inn" and others do not. Most patients check out without ever seeing the "Holiday Inn." There is no rule that a
mastectomy patient must filter through the self-help wing. So,
if a sweet, people-loving friend wants to practice a bit of her
trade, why penalize her? Why penalize us both?

Much ado about nothing, I decide, but still I feel like a
school child chastised by the principal. I fret a lot about how
this might affect Jane's job.

Despite my drugged condition—or because of it?—I am
physically strong. For the first time I am able to grip my pink
plastic washtub with both hands and maneuver it beneath the
tap for filling, and then to scoot it sideways onto my bathroom
countertop.

Great Scott, I'm using my right arm!

A protest streaks up my arm and across my chest. Again I
feel as if my stitches are ripping. Agrippa grips.

"I'm going to give myself my own bath," I swear, so determined that my teeth snap on every word.

It is eerie to soap my right upper arm and feel nothing; it is
dead to the touch.

The bath proves to be hard physical labor, and soon I am
gasping for breath. My bandaged chest won't tolerate bending.
My left hand is clumsy, unaccustomed to labor. The smallest
movement brings pain to my right arm.

Various spots that Jane scrubbed yesterday are beyond
my reach. I still am struggling with the washcloth when Louis
arrives, but I'm not at all tempted to beg his assistance. I'm
partly unwashed and I'm going to stink—and then that nit-
picking nurse will be sorry!

To tide me over till breakfast arrives, Louis fetches me coffee and juice from the kitchen. I decline the stroll—I am maintaining distance between me and the nurse.

Louis and I smooch a bit.

My breakfast tray arrives at last, and my spirits go thud. Allowed to choose my own food at last, I have ordered French toast and here it is—one slice. My stomach rumbles.

Breakfast, though scanty, revives my courage. After Louis leaves for his office, I venture down the hall where I weigh myself on the same scale used the day before my surgery.

115 pounds.

Exactly the same.

Subtract the weight of one breast, add the calories of hospital starches. . . .

Louis will take home as much wife as he delivered to the hospital, but with the pounds arranged somewhat differently.

AFTERNOON: I'm so settled into hospital routine that I can answer unblinkingly when a nurse inquires if I had "a nice b.m." What I haven't expected are fact-finding visits from the hospital staff. A young woman who apparently is the hospital "trouble shooter" asks for my judgment of her institution.

"Next time I'm going to order a double portion of French toast," I confide, letting her know by my grin and my cheerful tone that I'm not unduly upset by starvation.

She grins, too. "Portions are a problem."

"Oh, the portions seem just right, usually," I insist. "It's just that I'm a French toast freak. But listen, I really think the food is great!"

Astonishment carves her face.

I qualify, "I've done a lot better with the food since I've been allowed to mark my own menu. Which hasn't been long. When it was done for me, my diet was heavy on the starches."

We worry this flaw a bit, and she figures my early move to the "Holiday Inn" jammed the menu-marking processes.

She seems so sincerely to be soliciting my reactions that I tell her about the noisy night I spent upstairs—the nasal-voiced woman yelling at her deaf and senile mother. . . .

"We are considering changes in our open-visitor policy," she tells me.

Having won her sympathetic ear, I comment on my right-handed rooms. "I've had a mastectomy on my right side," I confide (as if she didn't know!), "and in both of my post-surgery rooms the telephone is rigged up on my right, with too short a cord to move to a table at my left, and the nurses' call button is on the right. . . ."

She should tell me to count my blessings, that there are *sick* people in this hospital who would trade their complaints for mine any day.

But she doesn't, because she is a compassionate woman, and being a woman, she understands the trauma of having a phone within arm's length but beyond possibility.

Do there exist in this world any left-handed hospital rooms?

On the heels of the "trouble shooter" comes a well-groomed woman who introduces herself as the head housekeeper. She asks my opinion on the cleanliness of her domain.

"Spotless!" I exclaim. "And the ladies who clean are so friendly and concerned. . . ."

She, too, is happy with me.

But again I affix a rider to my certificate of approval. "There's one thing—a thing nobody would notice unless she were flat on the bed and staring straight up at the ceiling. It's that fluorescent light fixture. In all three of my rooms, the plastic panel has been littered with dead bugs and dust."

She looks up and grimaces. "You're right!" Her astonishment is clear and so is her relief at being off the hook: "That's maintenance," she says. "That's their job. They're supposed to wash the panel when they change the light bulbs."

"Oh, they probably do," I assure her.

"I'll report this to maintenance," she plans.

I envision somebody in overalls, carrying a wrench, arriving any minute to bash my head, which I deserve.

I reflect on the two ladies' visits. How great to be in a hospital where the staff cares about my morale!

NIGHT: Weird thoughts assail me, sometimes, when I am alone. I read the Hemovac instructions and its bold-type, all-caps warning, DO NOT AUTOCLAVE. Since autoclave is not in my vocabulary, I worry a bit. What is it I'm not supposed to do?

Too, I mull over my operation, wryly and imaginatively, picturing various techniques of mastectomy in my mind's eye. Perhaps the surgeon lops off the breast as a woodsman fells a tree, sawing steadily across its base toward a notch on the opposite side. Or does he nip a bit off here, a bit off there, and work toward the center? Or does he begin at the nipple and slice layer by horizontal layer, down to the pectoral muscles, or perhaps to the ribs?

Well, however the heck he does it, it's been done to me. I can't seem to work up any rebellious steam. What's done is done. What's over is over.

I wonder if there is a correlation between the glamour of a breast and one's grief at losing it?

Wednesday, November 22

Six Days After Surgery

MORNING: I bore all comers with details of my restless, miserable night. Dr. Clarkly assures me I'll sleep when I need sleep; a nurse suggests that I swallow a sleeping pill at 8 or 9 P.M., so its effects will overtake me by bedtime; Dr. DeHaven wonders aloud why I refuse the pill he prescribes.

Well, because I'm scared of drugs. . . .

Dr. DeHaven is here to unplug my Hemovac, the flying

saucer that has trailed along with me for six days. I have watched its oozings graduate from blood-red to yellowish; and lately, there has been less liquid for the nurses to collect and measure.

He hovers over me.

"Will it hurt?" I ask, cowardly as always.

"A little," he replies, honest as always. And he adds, "Now the fun starts."

He peels off the tape which has steadied the tubes at their entry point to my body. Next he tugs out the tubes themselves— and the dear little things don't want to exit so they dig their heels against my insides, and I feel every millimeter of their journey.

A real drag.

Afterwards a small discomfort lingers.

Souvenirs that remain are two scars, smaller than dimes, which I suspect will be with me forever.

NOON: Complaining about the rancid odor of my chest, I am granted permission to shower. There are shower stalls in the rooms on my side of the hall in the "Holiday Inn," bathtubs across the way.

I covet a bathtub, but I'm stuck with a shower.

I twist the shower knob with my unschooled left hand, and I display great patience, but I am unable to gentle the gush of water. I don't dare let such a force beat on my incision. There is nothing to do but back my fanny into the harsh spray and let droplets ricochet. What I accomplish is merely a sponge bath with a change of scene.

My right arm remains a handicap, and by the time I towel myself dry, I am solidly fatigued. I must rest.

Up once more, I face the grooming necessity forced by Dr. DeHaven. He is a nut on underarm shaving.

With contortions, I manage to shave patchily under my left arm. But I bog down at the right armpit. Since there is absolutely no feeling beneath my right arm, I could slice myself open and never know it until I saw blood.

So I am a coward with the "safety" razor—and with reason. I have been warned to avoid injury to my right arm because its healing mechanism, the lymph nodes, were removed during surgery.

Can Dr. DeHaven seriously expect me to shave this dead-to-the-touch armpit?

REFLECTIONS: My company is spaced perfectly. There are enough visitors to keep my days from dragging but not so many as to tire me.

The bulk of them are women, of course. The men, when they come, seem embarrassed by my new handicap.

In an all-woman situation, the dialogue is predictable. Every single one of my friends asks, at first opportunity, "Did you find the lump yourself or did your doctor find it?"

I respond, "I found it myself, and it was a miracle, because I've never been diligent about self-examination."

"Oh, I'm not either," say my visitors.

One of my dearest friends exclaims, "Oh, I never do that!" as if it were the most odious chore imaginable.

So now I have a soapbox, and I warn that one woman in thirteen our ages faces breast cancer sometime in her life, as does one in eleven new-born baby girls.*

"But I don't know how to check my breasts!" I hear repeatedly.

Oh, how true! While printed instructions for self examination are available through American Cancer Society offices and from doctors, we women don't avail ourselves of this help. Or we do an incomplete job. Or a sporadic job. What we all need is personal supervision by our own doctors, watching while we prod our own breast flesh. We need on-the-spot

*These were the statistics in November, 1978.

instruction to build our confidence in our own detective work.

Just think: ten or fifteen minutes a month to save one's own life!

Busy physicians probably won't volunteer this instruction. We women must display enough gumption to demand the help we need.

AFTERNOON: I am going to get gorgeous for Thanksgiving! The same nurse who chastised me a few days ago has inveigled the ladies at the hospital beauty parlor to squeeze me into their pre-holiday schedule, with the agreement that I'll eschew rollers and settle for a bun at the top of my head.

Which is exactly how I've been wearing my hair this past fashionable week.

There is one difficulty. To my name I have exactly five dollars, the amount of cash suggested by the hospital on the day I checked in. So far I haven't spent a cent. (Ho, ho, Dorothy, don't forget the charges accumulating in the hospital business office!)

But my scalp itches and I can't lift my right fingers to scratch, so I decide to throw myself on the beauticians' mercy when the time comes to pay. I am under the dryer when a friend enters the shop, a true alien, a healthy and normal creature from the Outside World. The hospital beauty shop accepts nonresidents.

I borrow money from her.

Thanksgiving Day

One Week After Surgery

It is Thanksgiving morning.

During a therapeutic walk I meet a new "Holiday Inn" neighbor, Lucy, whose daughters and mine were high-school pals. We trade family news, then speak of our ailments. She has undergone gall bladder surgery.

I relate my astonishing lack of pain, my surprising emotional health.

"You're a brave woman," she praises me.

"Oh, no, I'm not! It's just a matter of priorities: alive with one breast or dead with two."

"You have a point," she concedes. But obviously, she wouldn't trade her malady for mine.

She is going home for Thanksgiving. So, it seems, are most of the patients. There is a threat of closing the "Holiday Inn" and transferring the few of us upstairs, which I would hate.

Hate!

Prowling the hall is an elderly woman who belongs to my "sorority." She wears our badge—the Hemovac. On her arm is a tight elastic "glove" to counteract post-mastectomy swelling, swelling I fortunately am not experiencing.

Apparently the glove is not worn overnight, and she confides that it takes all her strength to tug it on in the mornings.

How frail she is! I ache for her.

I ache more as her story emerges in bits and pieces. She first consulted a doctor about leg problems, mentioning in passing that her breasts were lumpy.

"He said to take care of that first," she reports. "So when I recover from this mastectomy, I'll have my second breast removed. And then I'll have operations on my knees, both knees, one at a time."

Oh, dear God!

Again I reflect on how kind God is being to me. My cancer is cut away. There is no spread of the disease. I am fine. *Thank you, God.*

For a holiday treat, Dr. DeHaven snips and plucks away half of my big black stitches. Pink lines remain where the stitches were, and sore red dots on my chest indicate each spot the needle entered.

On this holiday, the hospital is dreary. Only Louis comes to visit, and hours stretch long. Our conversation repeats yesterday's: the rude misbehaviors of Agrippa, and what is happening beyond my prison-like walls. There comes a point when Louis and I are boring ourselves and each other.

It is not a highlight of my day when a young trainee from the physical therapy department arrives to initiate my exercise program. How simple to lie lazily in bed and lift my right arm up and then across my chest!

Hah.

Simple it is not.

Painless it is not.

What it is, is *impossible*. My tennis elbow, my arm, my slashed chest all slam on the brakes.

Tears well in my eyes. "I never was good at calisthenics," I alibi.

"It takes time." She is being polite but, clearly, I'm not a prize pupil.

She teaches other cute little maneuvers to be performed in bed—or not to be performed, as in my case. Then she hustles me out of bed to a position facing the wall.

My defenses go up. I've been warned by mastectomy graduates about "climbing the wall." The idea is to start low and touch four fingertips to the wall, one at a time, each contact higher than the last. And to keep climbing until the brakes go on—and then to climb just a bit more.

"Every time you do the exercises, you'll go a little higher," the trainee promises.

I entertain doubts.

The mere straightening of my arm drills pain into my elbow. That doggone tendonitis.

I can't quit! I won't! Spunky by nature, I'm ready to fight. I can't go through life babying my right arm. As a left-hander, I am a klutz.

So what's so difficult about climbing the wall? I work at it. Lord, how I work! At chest level the brakes go on.

"I can do it," I lie. As my fingers start low and spider upward, I sing, "The teensy-weensy spider walks up the water spout."

The trainee doesn't laugh. Perhaps she never was a Brownie Scout. Perhaps she is right: this is no laughing matter.

So I shape up and concentrate totally, willing my fingers to creep. "How high am I supposed to go?" I wail.

She stands beside me and maneuvers her own fingers up, up, meanwhile walking toward the wall until her small nose touches it and her arm extends straight overhead.

I feel the stretch of her arm in my own belly, and a taste of vomit jumps to my throat. Fighting dizziness, I grasp a chair.

"I'll come twice tomorrow to help you with the exercises," she threatens.

"Happy Thanksgiving," I reply, without enthusiasm.

Louis eats hospital turkey and trimmings with me, I at the desk where I eat every "Holiday Inn" meal as per first-day instructions, he using a footstool as a table. When he returns home, our telephone is ringing.

It is my father.

We have decided to spare him the news of my cancer. As an eighty-six year-old widower living alone, he has enough burdens without adding concerns for my health and longevity.

"Dad, Dorothy isn't here," Louis admits. "I'll have her call you tomorrow or the next day."

Spared of worry about my health, my father no doubt can worry instead about the stability of my thirty-year marriage. Where could I be, if not at home on a holiday?

Friday, November 24

Eight Days After Surgery

True to her threat, the trainee comes morning and afternoon to supervise my agony of exercise. I am suspicious that I never will lift my arm again.

Well, no wonder! My upper arm is dead to the touch. My

side, below my armpit, is part dead, part tingly. I can't imagine the condition of my right chest; I'm not about to prod it to test it.

The trainee struggles with me. As an athlete, I am a flop.

But no matter. *I am going home!*

It is a home-going with strings attached: No sex for three weeks. Persistent exercise. An office call next Tuesday.

Before he releases me, Dr. DeHaven plucks the last of my stitches. I am happy to see them go.

The "Holiday Inn" nurse will inform us when my official release reaches her. Meanwhile, Louis and I go to the basement library, where we view the vidiotape of a young friend of ours, a male nursing student who had cancer of a salivary gland, a particularly fearsome cancer that threatens recurrence for thirty years.

Our friend has deep religious faith and a trust in medicine. With simplicity and sincerity, he tells of discovering his cancer, of his treatment and its side effects, of the appropriate needlepointed slogan presented by a friend: Never take your spit for granted.

Accompanying himself on the guitar, he sings two country-style songs that he has written about his cancer experience, and I watch through a blur of tears. Had this patient-performer been unknown to us, still I would have cried. But he is my friend, and he is too young for his life to be in jeopardy.

I hide my tears from Louis; perhaps he is hiding tears from me. We both are shivering. The projection room is stone cold, like a tomb.

We return to my room and finally, finally we are free to go. Out in the lobby, we encounter Mickey, who has come to give me various tips including the ins and outs, ups and downs, of prosthesis buying. She is impressed by the naturalness of available breast forms.

"You can't tell," she promises. "You really can't tell!"

I am grateful for her help and concern. And I am anxious to heal so that I can buy a prosthesis and continue on with my normal life.

Louis has washed our car for my homecoming; indeed, this is a red-letter day! Gingerly, but with great tenderness, he assists me into the car.

Then he slams the door.

Oh, my God! I am an eggshell beneath a hammer.

He gets behind the wheel and slams his door.

I gasp, "You've got—you've got to quit doing that!"

We stop at a drug store to fill a prescription for pain pills, "just in case." Of course this stop necessitates more car door slamming.

Certainly, my incision is split! Certainly, my ribs are crushed! When we reach home, I swallow a pain pill, partly to get my money's worth. (I was brought up by Germans who believed "Waste not, want not.")

Pretty soon, I go hoarse. My throat seems paralyzed. I barely can croak. In concern, Louis phones the pharmacist who suggests that the grain of codeine has relaxed my throat muscles.

This is relaxation?

The next time I need help, I swallow only one-half of a pill, and all is well.

Saturday, November 25

Nine Days After Surgery

All day, I lounge around in gown and bathrobe. I feel really crummy.

I have a peculiar mental block—I cannot remember the name of my operation. Repeatedly in the hospital I told people, "I had cancer, and I had a breast removed." That's calling a spade a spade!

But now I can't remember what that chopping off of the boob is called.

Louis consults the anesthesiologist's bill. "Radical mastectomy," he says.

"That's modified radical," I amend.

An hour later I can't remember the name of the surgery. Too bad I can't forget I had cancer.

As a fiction writer, my greatest plotting tool is a simple question, "What if . . . ?" Weird twists of plot emerge from this query.

Alas, today I am not keeping my professional life separate from my personal life. I am asking medical what-ifs that undermine my peace of mind.

What if the seeds of cancer escaped the breast and even now are dormant, waiting to blossom elsewhere? What if I lose my other breast? *What if I die too young?*

I recognize what I'm doing to myself, and I know the cure. To keep busy. I must involve my brain in urgent work, and when that fails, I must force my body to the point of exhaustion. I mustn't dwell on medical what-ifs.

In the days to come I force myself to bring this diary up to date. I write letters to be tucked inside Christmas cards. Unfortunately, neither of these diversions distracts me totally, because to grip a pencil still shoots pain all the way to my chest.

Pain or no, I work mountains of crossword puzzles. I bake cookies. Left-handed, I scrub moss from toilets. Diligently, somewhat panicky, I do my doggone exercises. Time is too precious to waste in brooding.

Sunday, November 26

Ten Days After Surgery

With Louis's help, I bathe and dress before breakfast, and I feel chipper all day. Well, chipper off and on. Friends tell me that my tiredness is the lingering result of the anesthetic, not of the surgery. However, I learn later that much blood is lost during mastectomy, the consequence of which is fatigue, until the blood rebuilds.

Monday, November 27

Eleven Days After Surgery

Delighted to be at home and useful, I go through wifely motions and serve breakfast to my husband. All of my reaching and lifting is, by necessity, with my left arm.

Louis warns, "Now, don't do anything foolish. Don't get into that bathtub until I can help you."

He plants the seed of fear, and I recoil at the idea of falling on my tender arm. I agree not to take an unattended bath.

I'm off pills, but I feel drugged. I can't gather my resources, even to give myself a sponge bath, although I know that getting washed and dressed would help my morale. I fritter away the day in a gown and robe.

My exercises put me through hell, without notable progress. When I "climb the wall," I cannot chalk a new mark on the paneling, because I am unable to reach higher than I did yesterday. I am blue with discouragement.

The young hospital therapist has warned me against stretching too far too fast. This is not a danger, because my body puts on its own brakes.

Cheer comes into my lonely day when Nona arrives. Because her live-in mother underwent a mastectomy, Nona knows exactly what my handicaps are, and what I need most.

"I'll comb your hair," she announces. So I don't look too witchy when Louis returns home from work, bringing gifts from the hardware store: a pully and rope, which he installs. Standing forward from the pully, and facing away from it, I am to tug down on the rope with my left arm in order to raise my reluctant right arm.

I work diligently, struggling for a non-jerky motion. Surprisingly this exercise feels good. I work with the rope in front of me, and, alternately, with the rope extended at my sides.

Also, Louis saws the bristle end from a broom so that I have a rod to grip with both hands. I start low and raise both arms together. Until, too soon, the brakes go on.

Tuesday, November 28

Twelve Days After Surgery

NOON: Ready to resume normal living, I make reservations at a mildly posh place and invite my friend Olga to lunch.

Of course, she must drive.

When she arrives to pick me up, I am not ready. Although I am a bath person, I have settled for a shower to eliminate the dangers of a slippery tub. Still wet, and wrapped in a towel, I answer the doorbell.

"I'll show you my brand new chest," I offer, and although she protests I bare my scar. "See, it's not so bad."

She averts her eyes. "No, it's not so bad." Her voice is choked.

Why does my surgery bother other people, when it doesn't bother me? It is I who had the cancer.

"Help me dress," I plead. "I can do it myself, but with help it goes faster."

Today I am going to be a modern girl and go braless. Dr. DeHaven has suggested that I pad an old brassiere with nylon hose until my chest is healed sufficiently to buy a prosthesis. But the bottom band of a bra crosses my raw Hemovac scars, and nylon chafes and burns my incision.

I slide on slacks and shoes. Olga eases me into a wild-patterned blouse with a big neckline bow, and into my Kelly-green blazer. Deftly, she combs my hair.

I look just great.

By chance, there is a multitude of people whom we know in the restaurant, and they all are aware of my surgery. In two's and three's, they come to our table, and I reassure them. "I feel wonderful," I brag. "The surgery isn't bad at all—it doesn't even hurt."

One visitor to our table isn't convinced. Patty, herself, underwent a mastectomy three years ago. She is astonished— almost horrified—that I'm "out in society" so soon.

"Take it easy," she urges.

Wouldn't it be perfect to mark this debut of mine with a martini before lunch? Indeed! But booze and drugs are an explosive mix, and mid-afternoon discomfort is by now a familiar pattern to me. I can't sneak past 2:30 P.M. without swallowing half of a pain pill.

So I do without the martini, and Olga does too, out of kindness to me.

AFTERNOON: At 4:30 Louis comes home to drive me to the surgeon's office. I could get myself there in a cab, but he wants first-hand information. Knowing how I despise calisthenics, he fears that I might bend instructions to my convenience.

I stand in Dr. DeHaven's examination room in my silly, open-down-the-front paper jacket. No bulge of breast blocks my straight-down view of my navy blue slacks.

Horrors! My slacks are white with dandruff-like specks.

"I'm molting," I say in embarrassment. "Is that from the penicillin?"

"Oh, no," he answers. "Your skin is flaking where the tape was."

Most urgent on my mind is the swelling beneath and behind my armpit. We women with this surgery tend to band together, and Kate, whom I had known only slightly, had generously come to the hospital to visit and commiserate with me. Her surgery had paved the path for me only two weeks earlier, and she was quick to tell me that twice already she had needed her armpit swelling aspirated—sucked out by a needle—a procedure which had been painful and frightening to her.

So I remember Kate's ordeal, and I brace myself.

The doctor compares one armpit against the other. "You don't have swelling," he decrees.

My relief is tremendous.

Still standing, I tell Dr. DeHaven about the knife-sharp

pains that slice into me, then ebb. I relate Agrippa's mischief. I mention the spot on my breast bone that restricts movement, a spot two inches beneath the lower end of my incision. "Why is the tightest pull way down there?" I wonder aloud.

Dr. DeHaven lifts my arm.

I rise on my tiptoes to alleviate the stretch.

"You're cheating," he accuses.

"I can't help it. You're hurting me."

Peculiarly, it is a good hurt. He knows the limits of my endurance.

He teaches Louis how to exercise my arm in the same way.

I have not been doing my home exercises adequately; the program of fifty daily movements to the point of pain, suggested by the hospital therapist, now is outdated. I am to exercise many times a day, and beyond the point of pain.

Tonight as I write this diary, my chest is aflame. I understand its anger; it has been maneuvered far beyond its will. Also, it has been outsmarted! Today I reach two inches higher than I reached yesterday. There is chalk on the paneling to prove it.

Wednesday, November 29

Thirteen Days After Surgery

I wish two things: I wish people wouldn't write me get-well notes that sound like rehearsals for sympathy messages to my family. And I wish the newspapers wouldn't print so many discouraging cancer articles.

Tonight our twelve-page local paper runs two banner headlines about cancer. The lead of one reads, "Two out of three cancer victims will die of their affliction."

Thursday, November 30

Two Weeks After Surgery

We are at breakfast.

"Are you really strong enough to go to the retirement party?" Louis asks, worriedly.

"Of course!"

"You'll have to be ready the minute I pick you up," he warns, since I hold no record for promptness even at the healthiest of times.

"I can do everything by myself," I brag. "It just takes a little longer."

Allowing plenty of time, I am about to back into the shower when Nona arrives. "What do you need?" she asks. "A haircomb? Dishes washed?"

I am overwhelmed by her repeat of last week's thoughtfulness.

So I have companionship, and it is Nona who dries my back, eases me into clothes, arranges my hair. . . . We compare my scar with her mother's more extensive radical surgery done in 1945 at Mayo Clinic. Her mother lived on for fifteen years and died at age ninety-one, without cancer recurring.

There are ninety people at the luncheon retirement party, and most of them give a speech, it seems. I am in trouble because every word spoken is funny, and how it hurts to laugh! Especially the bottom inches of my incision hurt.

Our retired friends, Rhonda and Rob, drive me home. It amazes me how thoughtful they are, insisting that I sit in the front seat while Rhonda crawls into the back of their two-door car. They even know beforehand that the slam of the car door will hurt me.

At my house, Rob rushes to open the car door for me, and Rhonda offers to help me change clothes.

People are astonishing! They anticipate my needs and are johnny-on-the-spot to help.

I brood over my sins of omission. I've sent cards and given gifts, yes, but I've never HELPED a sick friend.

DECEMBER 1978

Friday, December 1

Fifteen Days After Surgery

Louis is taking a day of vacation—a day we might have spent in Mexico with a little bit of luck.

From a sofa in our family room, I watch four squirrels frisk and leap and gnaw on hedge apples, those inedible (by humans) fruits of the Bois d'Arc tree. The squirrels are more humorous, joyous, and active than ever. What is the attraction of the chartreuse, grapefruit-sized fruits? Are they fermented?

Are the squirrels drunk?

In any case, I envy their pep and stamina. I seem to possess neither.

Saturday, December 2

Sixteen Days After Surgery

Today we drive a hundred miles to view an art film—my first out-of-town trip since surgery. In the crowd, I am protective of my right arm which remains numb and clumsy. The rest of me, praise the Lord, feels one hundred per cent normal.

Sunday, December 3

Seventeen Days After Surgery

I am washing my own hair! Both hands are working in unison—what a marvel of body engineering! I'm sudsing, scrubbing, rinsing. . . . This is a true landmark occasion.

For the first time, I am totally ignored by the rude Agrippa. He is taking Sunday off, refraining from sharply twisting my absent nipple, refraining from pinching my absent breast.

There is no phantom pain at all.

Monday, December 4–Friday, December 8

I am sentenced to five days of physical therapy because my progress displeases Dr. DeHaven.

The Physical Therapy Department is in a wing of the hospital. I lie on my back on a high bed in a windowless cell, while the therapist places hot packs on my right shoulder and around my trouble-causing elbow. The packs are bulky and moderately heavy. Almost immediately, their soothing and comforting warmth oozes deeply into my flesh.

Nestled at my ribs is a bell for ringing in case the gel-filled packs grow unbearably hot—and their temperature, indeed, seems to increase as minutes pass. I hit the panic button once or twice during the week but generally I tough it out, grateful for the heat and for the uninterrupted peace.

The small room is dark, and it is early afternoon: naptime. Day by day I relax more completely until, on Friday, I fall soundly asleep.

After I simmer for twenty minutes, the therapist returns to remove the hot packs and to soothe on lotion from my shoulder to my fingertips. This gentle touching is not without pain, but every stroke of an educated hand promises healing.

After the massage, the therapist lifts my arm and lowers it, lifts and lowers, all in a specific pattern designed to encourage my mobility. I am an antique automobile getting cranked, and not without discomfort. But I savor every minute! I feel the stretch: oh, so much farther than I can stretch by myself. I am encouraged.

In time, I am ordered to stand.

"Show me the exercises you do at home," I am told. It is important that I do them correctly.

Each day I learn something new.

Each day I progress, I truly do. This physical therapy is a great idea.

Wednesday, December 6

I have set my Wednesday appointment with Dr. DeHaven to follow immediately after therapy, when I am most agile; I'm not so dumb. This is the day he will decide if I can go on vacation—to the seashore of Florida, now, instead of to Mexico.

Louis suspects that I'll put words into the surgeon's mouth, so he accompanies me. He might as well; he's already on vacation. Some vacation.

I don't believe this right arm belongs to me! It is limber and mildly strong. It does me proud.

"Go!" says Dr. DeHaven.

By bedtime, I barely can move a muscle.

Thursday, December 7

Three Weeks After Surgery

Thursday again. The three-week anniversary of my surgery

and the 37-year anniversary of the Japanese attack on Pearl Harbor. A day for reflection.

My social life is destined to bloom! Because of my cancer operation, I have been invited to join Bosom Buddies, a local group of women who meet monthly for lunch. Membership requirement: a mastectomy.

Yesterday, Dr. DeHaven signed a permission slip for me to begin Encore, a nationwide YWCA-sponsored program for post-mastectomy women. The routine is a set one: exercises in the water, dry land exercises, and rap sessions. Locally the group meets once a week, directed by a nurse, who happens to be a tennis pal of mine.

Too, there is speculation that Reach to Recovery will be reactivated here. This is an organization which, upon request by the doctor, sends representatives to hospitals to visit mastectomy patients, to answer questions, and to be Exhibit A: "I, too, underwent mastectomy, and look at me now! Well dressed, brimming with vitality, and feeling fine. . . ."

Bosom Buddies.

Encore.

Reach to Recovery.

I shall be busy, indeed.

Saturday, December 9–Tuesday, December 12

Normally, I am a sentimental pushover for places that I love: I always ache to return. This time I feel differently. I yearn to explore a beach that is new to me, one to cling forever in memory, as my After-Cancer Beach.

We fly to Miami and rent a car, and we drive to Key Biscayne. We have no hotel reservations.

Surprisingly, there are few hotels on the key. We scout and make our choice.

We walk the beach, and our feet cake with tar. We eat expensively. We listen to palm trees rustle. I sleep a lot.

We love it all, but by Tuesday we are ready to move on, to familiar places.

Wednesday, December 13

I am in Miami Beach, and I am wearing my bikini.

My bikini!

The right side of my bra is stuffed with dacron, a gift from Christy. My chest above the bra is more flat on the right side than on the left. The red slash of my incision shows only a trifle, top and bottom.

These flaws are not open to view because a hotel towel is draped across my right shoulder. Dr. DeHaven has emphasized the dangers of sunburn.

We look out at the Atlantic Ocean from a terrace crammed with blue beach chairs. Those occupied are fitted with mattresses and umbrellas, but the majority are idle; this is the lull before the Christmas rush.

Even when I zip to my room on an errand I don't feel overly conspicuous, but upon my return a middle-aged woman calls to me as I pass her chair. "Do you know what you look like? You look like somebody about to burp a baby, with that towel over your shoulder."

I sit on the wooden slats of the chair beside hers and unload on her the entire tale of my cancer, beginning with my discovery of the lump last July, continuing right up to my bra-stuffing experiment this morning.

Asking questions, she is not feigning interest; she knows that she too might face breast cancer. Moreover, she is astute enough to realize that I need to talk at this precise minute, or explode.

"It's not so bad," I assure her. "In fact, I'm writing a book about it."

To unload on her benefits me, but I can't help wondering if I've cramped her natural friendliness forever. Will she ever again cast a casual comment toward a stranger passing by?

Thursday, December 14–Friday, December 15

Every day Louis rigs up the pully and rope from home and supervises my exercises. I am diligent, but I suspect that the Florida heat is helping as much as the tedious arm routines.

I still cry, sometimes, when I exercise.

At Miami Beach the hotel pool is heated, so on Thursday, when there is no audience, Louis exercises my arm under water. Magnificent! The buoyance of the water allows my arm new freedom to stretch forward and back, high and low. . . . I am doing great! Just think, only four weeks ago I was on the operating table.

On Friday I am sick. My chest is afire. My arm aches. I am so exhausted that my eyes barely focus. There is danger in exercising too little, I'm told. Also, there is danger in exercising too much, too soon.

Saturday, December 16

On Saturday, we drive up the Florida peninsula to visit my father in Clearwater. That is, Louis drives. The mere thought of maneuvering a steering wheel shoots arrows to my chest.

We should have flown. My aching body fails to fit the contours of the car seat. I fidget. I squirm. The journey seems endless.

In my father's yard, the flag is flying to celebrate our arrival, as it always is. A family tradition. My father greets me with a giant hug.

I scream.

"Are you getting a bit of arthritis?" he inquires as he loosens his arms.

I spin away from him, choking on sobs as I run. Behind a shut bedroom door I give way to fitful weeping. My body shakes. My teeth clatter.

This violent pain, like those before it, ebbs promptly. But I continue to cry nonstop. Oh, I am so tired! I am so worn from acting brave. Would that I could trade my cancer for "a bit of arthritis!"

Louis and I continue to conceal my surgery from my father. Why should we cause him concern over a situation that he can't change or control? To his generation, cancer equates with death. He might not believe that statistics are in my favor.

During our short visit, my father watches me move gingerly, favoring my right arm. He watches Louis pamper me even more than usual.

But he asks no more questions.

Friday, December 15–Friday, December 29

Five to Six Weeks After Surgery

Perhaps Agrippa prefers Florida to the southwest; he abandons me during my vacation and never again tweaks my lost nipple nor squeezes my missing breast.

Back at home, I continue to hate every moment of exercise, but I persist. There is a change in the nature of my pain while exercising. Before, there was impasse. Now, although the brakes still grip too soon, there is a hint that each stretch measures an iota of distance farther. Daily the chalk marks are higher on the wall. I'm making progress!

All the while, an annoying tightness remains in my upper chest.

In the morning, especially, I cradle my arm without realizing it. Then Louis reminds, "Swing it." But my arm is so much more comfortable when its weight is supported! Jealously, I reflect that some surgeons prescribe slings for mastectomy-affected arms.

Never do I slide backward. Improvements brought about by physical therapy hold fast. My tennis elbow is cured. Surely I can return to the tennis courts by spring!

I reach a milestone when Dr. DeHaven permits me to drive. (How it rankles that other of his mastectomy patients earn this permission much sooner!) Now I haunt the library. I have a compulsion to learn everything—everything!—about cancer.

I read technical reports. I read predictions. I read biographies of cancer victims who struggled for life and died bravely. I read autobiographies of those who made it—at least, long enough to commit their experiences to paper as I am doing. All this material is upbeat. As one title asserts, "The Climate Is Hope."

Not so upbeat is the deluge of recent material bad-mouthing mastectomy. Some "feminists" are on the warpath, demanding cancer treatment without what they call "amputation" of the breast. Doctors squabble among themselves and in the media as to the best procedure. Everybody is wishing it were possible to treat breast cancer without mastectomy, but doctors shy away from risking their patients' lives by employing procedures with ambiguous and patchy cure-rate statistics. A few bold doctors who have faith in non-mastectomy treatment, and a few women who refuse mastectomy, are pioneers. Years in the future, the statistics that they are building will become meaningful.

Even before the birth of Christ, medical chroniclers were reporting mastectomy as a treatment for breast cancer, an ordeal of intense pain before the discovery of anesthetics. In our time one name, William S. Halsted, is dominant in this field. It was in 1894 that Dr. Halsted published his mastectomy technique and observances, possibly jumping the gun on other surgeons doing similar work. Dr. Halsted's technique remained the prime way to combat breast cancer until the 1940's when the "modified radical" began to find favor among surgeons.

Halstead's procedure was to remove the breast, axillary (underarm) lymph nodes, and pectoral (chest) muscles. He retained only enough chest skin to close the wound; sometimes he purposely cut away so much skin that a graft was necessary. It was his goal to get rid of all body tissue which might conceivably host cancer.

The pectoral muscles are the push-and-pull muscles, and some women were handicapped greatly by their absence. Also the startling change in chest appearance—from fleshy bosom to cavity—created emotional trauma in many patients.

As years passed, surgeons discovered that they could reach and remove the lymph nodes without removing the pectoral muscles. This allowed the patient's arm to retain its push-and-pull ability. Her chest became little-girl flat, not hollow. This technique, called the "modified radical," produced survival rates substantially identical with those of the Halsted method.

While my research claims that the modified radical was accepted in the 1940's, I personally know of no mastectomee who received this milder surgery before the 1970's. Beginning in 1975, the modified radical mastectomy became the most frequent treatment for breast cancer in certain cases: when the tumor is located in one of the outer quadrants and is not attached to a muscle.

The reason that inner-quadrant cancers may necessitate muscle removal is that in this area the lympathic spread is through the muscle to lymph nodes behind the rib cage, near the breastbone. The cancer cells actually get a free ride inside the lymphatic vessels, through the muscle.

When the tumor is located in an inner quadrant, radiation usually is prescribed to kill any cancer that might remain after surgery.

To surgeons, mastectomy in many cases is less a "cure" than a staging technique to determine if further treatment is needed. In stage one, the cancer is in the breast only, in stage two it has spread to the nodes, in stage three the spread reaches beyond the nodes, and in stage four the cancer is widespread in the body.

A patient with widespread cancer is in immediate need of chemotherapy. Then the Halsted radical is eschewed and either a simple or a modified radical mastectomy is performed, or possibly no surgery at all. The goal is to initiate anti-cancer treatment rapidly.

In stages two, three and four, with cancer spread beyond the breast, treatment by radiation and/or chemotherapy is recommended not by one person's judgment but by the hospital's tumor committee composed of oncologists and surgeons. In our small city, which cannot support an oncologist, two internists sub-specialize in oncology and are specifically trained in the area of chemotherapy. They take part in the tumor committee's meetings, as do our city's three surgeons.

Despite the current popularity of the modified radical mastectomy, some surgeons still shun it, sincerely believing in the Halsted technique. Should a patient prefer the modified operation, she may have to seek another surgeon.

There exists a third technique, the "simple mastectomy" with or without implants. Only the breast is removed; pectoral muscles and lymph nodes remain in place. This surgery is used when a woman's breasts are so lumpy that biopsy after biopsy appears inevitable, or when a woman chooses to have a lumpy and suspicious second breast removed as a safeguard, her first breast having been cancerous.

Down the scale even farther are the "lumpectomy" and similar small surgeries in which only the cancer and some surrounding tissue are cut out. Radiation treatment follows the lumpectomy, and there have been some claims that when the lymph nodes are not involved (as in my case) survival rates are the same as with mastectomy.

Other records dispute this claim. Many more studies of lumpectomy patients are needed before statistics become trustworthy.

The great danger in both simple mastectomy and lumpectomy is that an undetected tumor might remain within retained tissue and flourish later, as happened to Yvonne. (See case histories.)

Writers in women's magazines tend to rant and rave

against mastectomy, but I cannot line up on their side. I harbor no regret at opting for modified radical mastectomy with its time-proven survival rate.

"It's the best hope," my own surgeon declares, and he has convinced me. I laugh at skeptics who suggest that surgeons recommend mastectomy because surgery, not radiology, is their bread and butter.

But I do not presume to dictate to other women. If life does not seem worth living without a breast, the greater gamble may be appealing.

Perhaps I'm crustier than some women. In my reading I am shocked to note that among mastectomy patients, twenty-five per cent consider suicide, thirty-six per cent increase their intake of tranquilizers, fifteen per cent solicit professional help for emotional problems, fifteen per cent booze more. . . .

I challenge Dr. DeHaven with these statistics.

"What I have seen in my practice," he replies, "is women who use mastectomy as a starting point, women who build more productive lives from this point forward."

So who is challenging whom?

Thursday, December 28

Six Weeks After Surgery

Today I buy my stuffer for my bra! But I must remember to be sedate and call it a "prosthesis."

"Don't you dread this?" Olga asks.

"Oh, no! Actually I'm looking forward to it." Another adventure along life's path.

Little do I know! Today ranks as one of the worst days in my life.

Louis takes a day of vacation to drive me to the nearest major city where a shop specializes in medical falsies of all sorts. Supposedly they handle "the cream." At least they are reputed to have the largest selection.

We are escorted to a tucked-away room where about twenty different prostheses are on display, each in its own box, complete with guarantee. I gasp at the variety. Fascinating! I had no idea. . . .

Here prostheses run the gamut from simple weighted blobs of plastic at about $50 (fifty dollars!) to a German paste-on model at 250 dollars. Some are tucked into a nylon slip-cover. Some are shaped perfectly round, some like a teardrop, a few like a squat boomerang. Some boast pink nipples; others are nippleless. Some are flat-bottomed to fit smack against the chest; others are hollowed out, as if the woman retains a breast of her own to fit inside it.

Some, gel-filled, are advertised to "move as the body moves." These must be guarded against punctures, to avoid leaks.

All of them feel, more or less, like flesh to the touch.

But they are so miserably heavy!

"These are large sizes," the saleslady tells us. "The larger the size, the heavier the prosthesis, just like the woman's own breast."

Falsies must be weighted; this I know. Picture, otherwise, a breast flying high when its owner reaches to a top shelf. Picture me on the tennis court, stretching toward a wayward ball. Alas, the weight is a necessary anchor; it holds the false breast where it belongs. It provides body balance, particularly for the heavy-breasted woman. It prevents backache.

But its allure definitely is minimal.

I pick three models, the lesser of all evils. Then I confront a plastic box of bras, size 36-A, and my heart sinks. Never have I seen such huge harnesses! There is enough fabric to sew a parachute. Pockets are sewn into the cups to secure the prostheses. The shoulder straps are three times wider than those to which I'm accustomed.

No adjustment can make the bra fit.

"I can't believe this!" I cry. "I've worn a 36-A forever."

The saleslady brings a box of 34-A's. They don't appear substantially smaller.

I wear one, and she tucks my chosen prosthesis into the pocket.

Wow, how buxom I am! The prothesis fills out the bra, but my own left side is woebegone.

"I can fix that," the saleslady announces.

Her "fix" is with a gel-filled falsie, the kind that "move with the body." Like its big brother, it is weighted and supplied with a hard core to simulate a nipple. It is less than one inch thick.

I am to wear it atop my own adequate, remaining bosom. *Dammit, I won't!*

So we try about every prosthesis in the shop, and a multitude of bras, and two hours pass. Two hours! All this time I am standing, until I am so weak I am ready to settle for anything, just to escape from there. Louis, too, is at the end of his rope, although he pretends patience.

We go back to the first arrangement, the number five prosthesis for the right side, the gel falsie for the left. With two bras, the cost approaches two hundred dollars.

"You'll get used to the weight," the saleswoman insists. "You are tired now, and weak from recent surgery."

About that, she certainly is right. What she doesn't guess is that my healing chest is screaming its rebellion. It has endured two hours and twenty minutes of chafing and abuse.

I refuse to wear the expensive contraption home.

New Year's Eve

My debut with my prosthesis is to be made at a neighborhood New Year's Eve party. I am excited! I want to strut a bit, to show off my rapid recovery. I want to be the Grand Dame of Bravery.

I choose a semi-clinging dress, all the better to show off my newly purchased bosom.

But nobody looks at my chest. In fact, nobody even mentions my operation. I don't bring it up, of course, but I want to! I still need to talk about it, perhaps to dispel the Ghosts of Cancer Past.

JANUARY 1979

Thursday, January 4

Sleet has iced our hills and I am housebound, a condition to which I react badly because I am a seashore girl. A *tropical* seashore girl. Listlessly I wander around the house, wondering why the phone doesn't ring (has the world forgotten me?), too lethargic to call out. Besides, to dial the phone still drills pain straight to my chest.

I could invite neighbors over to break this monotony, but I can't stir myself to do so.

In my wanderings, I remind myself that I am free to do absolutely anything I please. Anything! The indulgence is mine because I have had cancer—should my years be numbered, it is essential that I enjoy every minute now.

Enjoy? How can I, when I am so sluggish and dull? I fritter away hours with jigsaw and crossword puzzles. I keep this diary, but I make no effort to reread and polish what I have recorded, nor do I query editors. This inefficiency is not in character; never before in my life have I knowledgeably wasted time.

I drag myself to bed mid-mornings and mid-afternoons and sleep soundly, but no quantity of sleep conquers my sluggishness.

Rare moments when I'm impelled to do housework, I force my right arm to action, as if it were a naughty child who needs discipline.

Discipline is big in my life; I still lean hard on my moral fiber in order to exercise. Miraculously, my right hand now "walks the wall" as high as the left; the chalk marks on the paneling have reached their zenith.

Their zenith, that is, when I exercise facing the wall. When I stand at right angles to it, interior brakes still restrain my fingers from climbing far.

Toward evening as I wait for the day's brightest moment, Louis's return home, my arm grows more and more leaden and relief comes only by propping it shoulder high on pillows.

Sunday, January 7

I am not wearing my prosthesis, not only because it chafes and burns my still-tender chest, but because of its weight. It is unbearably heavy.

I hated it the day I bought it, I hate it today, and I'll hate it until I die.

Oh, the constant misery of straps digging into shoulders! How do heavy-breasted women tolerate this punishing pull? Perhaps their shoulders aren't as bony and unpadded as mine.

Wearing the prosthesis, I feel as if I'm tilting forward. If I fall, I won't bump my nose, that's for sure! It is no consolation that I have the best bustline of my life. Now more than ever, I need to be ME. It is more and more apparent that my prosthesis is a misfit.

Wednesday, January 10

Git-up-and-go is smashing into me full force. Overflowing with energy, I am house cleaning and entertaining.

Christy is unsurprised. It takes six weeks, she claims, before a surgery patient feels normal.

I am writing, too, a lucky thing because this week I have

been offered a book contract based on two chapters plus outline. There is a deadline, so I have a chore ahead.

I get with it.

After typing on an electric machine for half an hour, hard-hitting pains arrow into my right ribs, into my chest wall, into my upper arm.

Louis urges, "Pay no attention. Dr. DeHaven says you can't hurt yourself."

My husband doesn't care that I hurt! He doesn't care!

Of course, I know he cares; I know he's hurting, too. So why doesn't he say so? Psychology stinks. What I crave today is pity.

Friday, January 12

My curiosity about my cancer is a fire that banks higher and higher. I consult every possible source, human and printed. During my surgical checkup, I ask questions from a prepared list—oh, poor Dr. DeHaven! He remains courteous and patient, and I learn a lot.

When my reading confuses me, I phone Christy for an insider's view of the hospital laboratory. It was in her lab, after all, where my "lump" officially was labeled cancer.

It was suspected to be cancer when Dr. DeHaven first cut into it, because it was "gritty," and because it had sent out "feelers" to adjacent tissue.

I continue to question until I piece together a picture of what happens to a breast cancer patient in the operating room. First there is the biopsy, the lifting out of the lump and some adjacent tissue, material which is carried on gauze to a table, away from the operating table. Here the medics examine what they are dealing with, and remove with a scalpel what they wish to study further.

In the laboratory, the sample is blown with carbon dioxide in order to freeze it, to enable it to be sliced more thinly—

exactly as I freeze raw pork and beef for thin slicing, for Oriental recipes.

Then an instrument called a microtome is used to cut tissue extremely thin, for microscopic examination. Thus prepared, the slices are "run through" a stain. On the stained tissue, trained persons can spot a typical cell pattern of cancer.

Christy comments that when a pathologist enters the lab with one of these lumps in gauze, the surgeon often is walking right behind him.

If the verdict is cancer, the operating room is "regrouped," anesthetic and equipment made ready. Then, apparently, the surgeon slits the skin on the "incision line," lays the skin back with "retractors," and lifts out the breast tissue in a process called "dissecting it out."

Dr. DeHaven is amused that I am compelled to learn all this. Also, I learn much more, bits and pieces. I learn that the "frozen sections" done between biopsy and mastectomy are only the start of the laboratory work. Permanent sections are prepared later, and filed at the hospital.

By now I am aware that breast lumps differ, one from another. There is the cyst, a fluid-filled marble that can be shoved around, and can be aspirated in the doctor's office, for laboratory testing.

Opposed to the cyst is the tumor, which is hard. My "cigarette stub" was a tumor. That it was anchored too firmly to be wiggled was a bad sign, not the good one I had imagined.

Thursday, January 18

Bosom Buddies meets for lunch, this month, at a long corner table in the local pancake house. There are about fourteen of us, half of whom I knew before my surgery.

I am comfortable right away. This is a relaxed group, a jolly group, linked by a common medical experience.

Bosom Buddies is social. Founded by three women who needed each other's encouragement during cancer treatment, the group expands to gather in novices like me. Because these women walked our path, and survived, our route is less shadowed with the terrors of the unknown. They are our models!

I wail my disenchantment with my prosthesis.

"You're much too tiny for a size five!" I am told. "Size five is much too heavy for you."

"I wear a size zero," Sarah tells me, quietly. She isn't a lot smaller than I.

I know I will have to make a change; I will have to be fitted again.

The ordeal looms like a mountain.

Saturday, January 20

Needing a change of scene, I take advantage of an art tour by bus to a major southwestern city. Between museums I go to a famous department store and inquire about prostheses.

In a wink I am fitted with a bra—my pre-surgery size, 36-A—and a prosthesis. Nothing to it! Oh, why had my first fitting required two hours, twenty minutes?

I buy the bra for nine dollars, exactly half the price of my other new ones. But I am gun-shy about prostheses, not trusting my judgment, not wanting a $120 disaster so soon on the heels of my $130 mistake.

Mail order is possible. I carry home the clerk's name.

But I procrastinate and never complete the transaction.

Tuesday, January 23

I ache all over, especially across my shoulders and at my upper spine. Is this from sitting cramped for hours in the bus? Is it a delayed effect of surgery?

I suspect, alas, I have brought the pain on myself by being overprotective of my purple, puffed, tender incision. Since my operation I haven't done my customary neckrolls or toe touching, much less my yoga stretching. My body begs for more than the mastectomy exercises that I perform so diligently and so joylessly.

Yet, I'm fearful that I'll pull something loose, some vital stitch or patch inside my chest.

So I ache.

Monday, January 29

For several years Louis and I have been trying to get into a CPR class, and now our turn arrives.

Cardiopulmonary resuscitation is not all theory; we practice on a dummy. I feel some chest discomfort when I force my breath into the dummy's mouth; I feel severe strain as I rhythmically push the dummy's chest.

I fear overstraining myself, so I tell the nurse in charge about my recent surgery.

"Did the doctor say you could do this?" she asks, worriedly.

"He said I can do anything. He said nothing can hurt me."

I'm doing CPR; I'm not doing yoga. I recognize my inconsistency.

Wednesday, January 31

At the all-day Reach to Recovery meeting, our out-of-town teacher encounters rebellion. Always before, she has addressed groups of individuals who were strangers to each other. Not so here! Bosom Buddies more seasoned than I hold firm opinions on how to help mastectomy patients, and some of these opinions conflict with the official Reach to Recovery edicts.

For instance, RR volunteers are banned from calling on any mastectomy patient in the hospital without an official request from her doctor, no matter how close a friend that patient might be. It is suggested among ourselves that the teacher is more concerned with protecting her organization from the possible wrath of surgeons than in the welfare of individual patients.

Three of us at the meeting aren't even supposed to be here since RR volunteers must be two years post-surgery. Two years to moderate the shock—or a buffer of two years, in case of cancer recurrence? A volunteer hardly can dish out hope if she knows her own cancer is spreading.

FEBRUARY 1979

Wednesday, February 7

I can't tolerate any more cancer talk, any more cancer thought: mastectomy meetings, mastectomy exercises, and my own extensive mastectomy research suddenly squash me. Too, I begin to debate my participation in Encore, the YWCA-sponsored program for post-mastectomy women, which combines swimming pool exercises, dry land exercises, and a let-your-hair-down rap session. Would I do better to put my head in the sand and forget the whole thing?

The nurse who directs Encore notices that my right shoulder is higher than my left, the result, she claims, of my going braless for three months.

"But my prosthesis is too heavy," I wail. "I hate it!"

After her scolding, I promise to wear the bulky, obnoxious harness for my own good. It is a promise I won't keep.

Wednesday, February 21

Three Months After Surgery

A psychologist is invited to speak at Encore, but she hardly gets a word in edgewise. The ladies vie with each other to describe, for her, the psychological effects of mastectomy. The heat generated is fantastic. Later, I tell the would-be speaker, "Introverts don't get breast cancer."

It is from this psychologist that I learn of yet another research book, "The Breast: Its Problems—Benign and Malignant—and How to Deal with Them" by Oliver Cope, M.D. I study it as I study others, but this particular book kindles doubt and distress, and undermines my optimism. It is Cope's statistic-supported claim that a breast cancer victim has only a fifty per cent chance of survival, the same whether or not her breast is removed. So, he suggests, why undergo the shock of mastectomy and possible handicap to arm and shoulder, when a small surgery followed by X-ray and/or chemotherapy produces equal results?

I rage against his statistics. I, for one, am promised an eighty-five per cent chance because my lymph isn't involved.

Louis, too, reads this book and others, and wonders aloud if we are leaving stones unturned. Unlike my Bosom Buddies, I have undergone neither bone scan nor liver scan, tests deemed unnecessary by local doctors. *Is their judgment correct?* Or should I seek further opinions from specialists at a major cancer clinic?

Am I playing Russian roulette with my life?

I understand the doctors' premise: that if my underarm lymph nodes are uninvolved, the cancer has not spread. Unfortunately, I am undermined by knowledge gained in research, and I know that although breast-cancer cells commonly are filtered by the lymph nodes in the axilla, they also might escape that filter and travel instead through the blood or through other sections of the lymphatic system. Then they are free to root and spread. Such knowledge is not soothing.

It is only natural, I suppose, that from time to time I fear the very worst for myself. Why else am I bleeding between periods, a symptom that started after the mastectomy?

I undergo tests, wait three nervous days for results, and then learn from my gynecologist that all is normal. I'm spared once again!

Thank you, God.

Now, three months past surgery, I am more fearful of cancer than I was as a patient in the hospital. I am drained of energy, and my optimism is shaky.

I pull myself up short. Don't I feel exactly this way at the tail end of every winter? I do.

Blame the weather.

MARCH 1979

Wednesday, March 7

Don't ever think that the gentle Encore exercises cause no pain! I feel a not-unpleasant stretch while doing them in the YWCA class—moderation is urged—but afterward the "trauma" to the pectoral muscles shoots complaints to me for days.

Of course I'm supposed to continue the exercises at home, daily. I'm fairly trustworthy in this department, but no longer 100 per cent diligent. I'm over the hump, I feel. I'm getting lazy.

Dr. Clarkly, my internist, adds to my knowledge and peace of mind. From him I learn that six months past surgery, three months from now, I will have a chest X ray. This X ray will indicate whether scans or other follow-up tests are needed. And I am to have a new mammogram annually, despite false negative readings of the past.

And monthly, of course, I am to examine my own breast for tissue changes. For early detection of recurrence, the responsibility is mine.

Sunday, March 18

Four Months After Surgery

I must be boring Louis out of his skull! To our evening hash-over of the day's events I bring only cancer-related news, an item in the press or a report from a Bosom Buddy.

For instance I learn from Teresa, three months my senior in terms of surgery, that she still wears a tight "stocking" on her arm to combat swelling, and that she spends a lot of time with her arm upraised. Without lymph nodes, the arm does not drain as before.

My recovery is easier.

Plus, I haven't needed cobalt.

Plus, I haven't needed chemotherapy.

I am thanking God in a way that surprises me, by worshipping in a church not my own. Here it is the custom to praise God on one's knees and to approach the altar rail for Communion. On my knees I am physically uncomfortable but emotionally tranquil. I sense the nearness of God.

Thursday, March 22

What caused my cancer?

If I could solve this riddle, the world would bow at my feet. The sad fact is, we just don't know what causes breast cancer. Maybe we never will know.

But I am a captive of my own inquisitiveness, and I must

ponder this question. I must seek clues. What was it about my body or my lifestyle that provided a fertile host for cancer?

Right now I am in the highest risk group for new breast cancer, having previously hosted the disease. But what contributed to my first cancer?

I contemplate some known risk factors, one by one.

1. A sister, mother, father, aunt, or grandmother with breast cancer. (I had none.)
2. A woman who has never given birth, or one who first gave birth after age thirty, or one who had an aborted pregnancy before eighteen. (I fit here; I never gave birth. My children are adopted.)
3. The use of estrogens, female sex hormones, for any of many reasons. (These never have been prescribed for me.)
4. A history of benign breast disease, encompassing various "lumpy" conditions. (Fortunately, I never developed the common fluid-filled cysts that doctors drain with needles, but I do indeed have lumpy breasts.)
5. A long reproductive period: early menstruation and/or late cessation of menstruation. (Guilty again. I continue to menstruate regularly.)
6. Obesity. (Not me!)
7. A relatively high position on the socio-economic ladder. (Many American women fit in this category, particularly compared with women in less developed countries.)
8. Overuse of X rays. (I have undergone no treatments with X rays, but over the years I have had many X rays for diagnostic purposes.)
9. Hypothyroidism. (Having swallowed three grains of thyroid daily since my teen years, I should not be at risk.)
10. Under suspicion: the use of hair dyes. (Guilty. Hopefully this danger is past because suspected cancer-causing ingredients have been removed from dye formulae.)

11. Under study: Diet. Seventh Day Adventists, who eat no meat, and Mormons, who restrict meat consumption, develop less breast cancer than the general population. Animal fats and proteins are highly suspect at this writing, and research continues. (There was a time that I fed my family meat three times a day, obeying the nutritional dictates then in style. Certainly over the years I have enjoyed vast quantities of steaks and roasts, the "red meat" my upbringing decreed as essential to my good health.)

12. Under suspicion: A virus which possibly roots and multiplies in a breast nourished by blood that contains an excess of female hormones.

13. Under suspicion: An ingredient in calorie-free and low-calorie soda. (I drank one or two cans per day during the two years prior to my mastectomy.)

14. A likelihood: Attitudes of hopelessness and despair. (These feelings certainly were not present to undermine my body's resistance to cancer.)

15. Under suspicion: Stress. Increased quantities of hormones are secreted during stressful times, and cancers do seem to emerge after family upheavals. (I was never immune from normal family worries, and my mother died at Christmas 1977, eleven months before my mastectomy.)

16. My own unscientific, unproven, and doctor-denied theory: Bras with underwires. (I had worn this style only one year before surgery, and where the wire bit my flesh was exactly where my cigarette stub of a cancer grew.)

17. Always a consideration: Something in the air. (Our small city is relatively pollution free, but we in the southwest battle cockroaches, and the spray used twenty years ago by a professional company remains effective in my home. I understand this particular chemical has since been banned.)

I mull these seventeen causative possibilities, and I concede how very receptive my body must have been to cancer.

Friday, March 23

I note with appreciation that the seven warning signs of cancer can be arranged so that their first letters spell *caution.*

1. Change in bowel or bladder habits
2. A sore that does not heal
3. Unusual bleeding or discharge
4. Thickening or lump in breast or elsewhere
5. Indigestion or difficulty in swallowing
6. Obvious change in wart or mole
7. Nagging cough or hoarseness

Saturday, March 24

With cancer too much on our minds, Louis and I need a change of scene. We grasp at an opportunity to spend a week in New York City.

At Chicago, where we change planes, I telephone Ursula who has written me a strong cheer-up message (not that I was uncheery) complete with news of her mastectomy eighteen years ago.

Ursula? A mastectomy?

This I never suspected although the two of us spent a beautiful day together baking on a beach. What I do recall is her modest swim suit.

So from now on, people will peg me as modest, not necessarily as breastless. But who cares, either way? I'm not going to quit going to the beach.

Sunday, March 25–Tuesday, March 27

It is Sunday, and Louis and I are playing tennis.

I am in seventh heaven. I knew I could do it!

Louis walks to the net and accuses, "You're wearing your arm band."

"If I don't wear it, I get tennis elbow." I cringe at memory of the pain.

Louis looks solemn. "You have instructions not to have your blood pressure taken on your right arm. You pull that band so tightly it leaves welts. It's as tight as a blood-pressure sleeve, and you leave it on an hour and a half at a time, or two hours. . . ."

He is right.

The bottom drops out of my world. So far I've been a soldier, but if my mastectomy robs me of tennis no telling what will happen to my mental health.

I'll be irritable, at the very least.

Under Louis's watchful eye, I remove the band and continue hitting the ball, but it isn't a true test because very soon he decrees, "Enough for the first time."

There is an ominous pinch in my elbow.

On Monday Dr. DeHaven says that if I can't play tennis without the arm band, I can't play tennis at all.

During four months of staunch bravery, I have stored a bushel of tears. Today I spend them all, weeping in anger, weeping in self-pity, weeping just for the luxury of it. But by evening the sun breaks through my cloudy skies. I see some hope.

The next morning I take a tennis lesson, the theory being that if I hit the ball correctly, tennis elbow won't be a problem.

APRIL 1979

Wednesday, April 4

My Bosom Buddies are, as the saying goes, "something else." Never have I belonged to a group so knowledgeable and clear-headed, yet optimistic. Faith and courage keep these women going, full speed ahead, damn the torpedoes.

Quickly I discover that I'm not the only patient who left her modesty behind with her breast flesh in the operating room. All of us are motivated by a show-and-tell philosophy. If our scar or our prosthesis or our "reconstruction" can impart information, we whip up our blouses.

Before I joined this elite group, I linked the word *reconstruction* with the era following the War Between the States. Now "reconstruction" means a silicone implant.

Victoria couldn't escape her mirror and its mocking reminder, "Cancer! Cancer!" With her reconstruction she again feels normal, again feels happy. She probably will skip a second step, the creation of a nipple.

Yvonne possesses a reconstructed nipple on a reconstructed breast. When she faced double mastectomy at age thirty-seven, she informed the doctors that her breasts were very much a part of her sex life and she refused to wait the recommended year for reconstruction. She won the battle, only to lose one of her new breasts as cancer recurred.

When in her 40's, Wanda underwent double mastectomy and suffered eighteen months of pain, her severed nerve endings snarled with scar tissue. Part of the surgeon's remedy was to cushion the painful area with implants, a technique with cosmetic side affects. Indeed, Wanda appreciates her rebuilt breasts—but she would not have opted for the surgery on an elective basis.

Wanda, that's how I feel! I don't want breast reconstruction. What I want is a face lift.

Monday, April 16

Five Months After Surgery

My continuing symptoms are so mild that I have to dredge deep to paint Dr. DeHaven a picture of my progress. "My arm still gets tired toward night," I report, "and I prop it on pillows. Is that all right?"

He nods.

I go on. "Some days there are lots of pins and needles in my arm and chest, and some days almost none. There's life coming back into the numb areas."

"Are you going to Encore?" he asks.

"Yes. And I'm playing tennis—without the armband. And I'm doing everything I ever did."

"Your discomfort will be less because you are active," he approves.

I pry out of him that some women suffer discomfort for five or six years, if not forever.

"I'll tell you one thing," I warn. "If I have to go through this again, and lose the other breast, I'm not going to be a model patient! I'm going to wail and rant and make everybody miserable."

His nurse laughs, as if I'm joking.

I'm not joking.

Dr. DeHaven believes me. He bows his head and the spring sunlight, so clear and harsh as it slashes through his window, illuminates the gray in his hair.

Gray! How has he advanced from a fifteen-year-old gangly youth to a mature man of my generation, in just five months?

In his new maturity it seems natural that he should inquire of my prosthesis, and I report on my new one, a 105 dollar blob of silicone encased in flesh-colored nylon. My original prosthesis cost 130 dollars.

Warmed to the subject, I relate, "The first fitter just eyeballed me, but this one used a tape measure and switched me from size five to size two. What a difference in weight! Now I can walk without tilting forward.

"But still it chafes," I complain. "And if I wear it more than a few hours at a time, it burns and stings against my healing chest. Doctor, is it really true that if I don't wear a weighted prosthesis, I'll get a backache?"

"Not you," he promises. "That is a problem of large-breasted women."

Rejoice that I'm small!

As I lie on his examining table, he prods my nice left breast and then my funny flat side.

"I have no confidence I'm self-examining properly," I confide, demonstrating how I do it.

"Use the flat of your fingers rather than your fingertips," he instructs. "Rock the flesh around."

"Like this?" I can't get the hang of it.

"No, like this." His fingers press mine into my breast. "See, here's a lump."

Here's a lump! How casually he says the dreaded words.

Indeed, he has located a tissue shockingly similar to my "cigarette stub" of a cancer. It is at three o'clock.

I stare at the ceiling, which is not in focus, and I ask quietly, "Well, what do we do about it?"

"At worst we'll have to biopsy it," he says.

Worst, bunk! There is something much worse than biopsy. It's the whole show, repeated, and a renewed worry about cancer.

He reminds, "The breast isn't two glands, but one. If lumps develop in one, they are likely to develop in both."

"Marvelous," I lie.

"We'll watch it," he promises. "Come back in three months."

Until today I have titled this diary "Mastectomy Without Tears." Today the title must be changed. I weep because I am sorry for myself, and I weep because I am angry.

I debate shielding Louis from this crummy news, but I can't. I need his support. Darn it, I need his sympathy!

So I share this tidbit from my day.

"WATCH IT!" he roars. "WAIT THREE MONTHS! We'll

do nothing of the sort! We'll go to M. D. Anderson. We'll go to Sloan-Kettering. We'll go to Mayo's."

He seems on the verge of packing our suitcases.

I don't want to go anywhere. I want to savor my promised three months, away from all doctors.

We compromise with my promise to consult Dr. Clarkly, who has been my internist for nearly thirty years.

Tuesday, April 17

To arm myself with information before my appointment with Dr. Clarkly, I phone Zita, a Bosom Buddy who is a registered nurse.

I tell her, "Louis can't figure out why Dr. DeHaven isn't going to biopsy immediately."

"The necessity for such speed has been disproved," she tells me. "Many, many women get cysts which are watched to see if they go away. You can't biopsy every bump that shows up."

Then she spoils her level-headed, non-emotional medical report by adding, "I know exactly how you feel! My remaining breast has lumps, too, and my doctor is watching them."

She is as nervous as I am.

Enlightened by Zita, I am unsurprised when, after his examination of me, Dr. Clarkly agrees with Dr. DeHaven's waiting game.

"I'm sure Dr. DeHaven merely wanted to show you what fibrous breast tissue feels like," he consoles me. "Now that you can locate it, you can check it—but don't go poking at yourself more than once a month."

"I know," I say.

How sheepish I am! I have wept for twenty-four hours, an exercise in futility. How many false panics does this make?

I'm a ninny! I must quit borrowing trouble.

JUNE 1979

Seven Months After Surgery

How will I feel, now, when long-time friends undergo mastectomy? Before my own operation I grieved for my friends, and nearly buried them.

Audrey returns from an out-of-town hospital, and I'm put to the test.

"Welcome to the club!" I tell her over the phone.

She is fantastic! Her spirits are high, she praises her doctors and her hospital, and she looks forward to chemotherapy with no fear.

Physically as well as mentally, she seems on top of the problem. She even set her hair the second night after surgery.

I applaud her, admitting, "I couldn't even lift my arm for weeks!"

To my surprise, she rejects invitations to Bosom Buddies and Encore although she is a socially-oriented person. Her plan is to follow her surgeon's instructions and otherwise to live as she always has, without outside reminders of cancer.

This is what she wants, so I support her. But I worry. Is she hiding from the truth?

JULY 1979

Eight Months After Surgery

My eighth-month checkup with Dr. DeHaven, my surgeon, indicates that my incision is healing normally and that, more important, my remaining breast is free of frightening symptoms. My own fingers no longer locate a "rope" at three o'clock.

AUGUST 1979

Nine Months After Surgery

Louis is studying at Stanford University and, as an offshoot, I am attending a class on problems faced by executives' wives.

I can't believe myself! A talker by nature, I sit silent while women report on traumas that they experienced when their husbands suffered heart attacks. It is so clear to me that the healthy partner suffers more than the sick person, and probably I should contribute this nugget of earned wisdom to these women who are distressed. Truly I believe my surgery was harder on Louis than on me.

But I no longer need to shout, "Look at me! I had cancer, and now I'm fine!"

My modesty is seeping back.

SEPTEMBER 1979

Ten Months After Surgery

The waiting room is the same, complete with *The Wall Street Journal*. The X-ray room is the same, but the technician's technique differs. This time my breast is sandwiched between the X-ray plate and clear plastic.

At the first failure, the technician says I must have moved. At the second failure, she admits that the developing paper went in wrong and the machine "ate it up." Three times is a charm—but I do worry about all that X ray bombarding me.

Dr. Pelt, my original radiologist, meets me in the examining room.

"Remember that 'normal breast tissue' you examined a year ago July?" I greet him.

Under my quizzing he admits a fifteen per cent failure rate for mammograms, divided about evenly between false negatives and false positives.

Why didn't anybody tell me this before?

I dig for more information. "I've read that even a pinpoint of cancer shows up on a mammogram."

"Not a pinpoint, but we've found them the size of the head of a kitchen match."

"I've also read that pathologists can mis-identify cancer."

"Not our boys!"

I'm glad that the doctors have faith in each other.

Once again I pursue the matter of my dense breasts. This time Dr. Pelt explains that at about age forty most women's breast tissue turns fatty. Mine has not done this, so last year's mammograms showed no difference between the breast tissue and the cancer. That is, my cancer hid itself.

Today my mammogram is, once again, negative.

Can I believe it?

OCTOBER 1979

Eleven Months After Surgery

I happen to be visiting in a major city when an elite store sponsors a prostheses promotion. Because I never have been satisfied with my second "breast form," I'm delighted at the opportunity to try again.

The fitter from company headquarters works hard to choose the right bra for me, then offers only one size of prosthesis. "This is the correct one," she insists.

I trust her.

At home I obediently sew a "pocket" in the bra to secure the prosthesis. How great the whole contraption looks and feels when I am standing tall!—as in the elite store's fitting room. But when I bend over to make the bed—ouch!—the stiff lower edge of the form knifes into my flesh. Also, it pokes me when I slouch. What's more, its weight seems to rest on my tender chest; the weight should be suspended, I think, from the bra's shoulder straps.

By noon the lower edge of the prosthesis has raised welts on my chest.

Did the "specialist" misfit me? Or is the stiff backing a flaw in design? I'm too blue to care. All I know is that once again, a "falsie" has been untrue to me. Goodbye 130 dollars.

NOVEMBER 1979

Friday, November 16

One Year After Surgery

One year is past! I am alive! And I feel wonderful.

Gazing backward twelve months, I judge myself with a clear eye, seeing myself fearless before surgery, brave afterward, and foolish in the stretch. How much anguish and worry we might have avoided, had I not mistranslated doctors' words, had I not ferreted out loopholes to my predicted recovery, had I not panicked about that rope at three o'clock!

From association with Bosom Buddies, I have developed The Abbott Theory of Mastectomy: It is not the amputation of the breast which haunts us, it is the very real, red flag of danger, the notification that we are mortal. How we handle this news-that-isn't-news is a gauge of our happiness.

How am I doing? Oh, splendidly! One proof is that when I bathe, I scrub my flat, right chest without even thinking about it, exactly as Ursula promised. My internal twinges of healing are ended. When I shave my armpit, there is some sensation to guide the blade so that I no longer risk suicide for cosmetic purposes. Numbness in my arm is eased; when I scratch, I feel my fingernails on my flesh—although scratching does not bring the same satisfaction as it did before surgery, because my upper arm retains a bit of its dead-fish stupor.

What is with me forever, I fear, is my chest and arm's tendency to tighten if I skip my daily arm-movement exercises.

To the eye, my incision is not unpleasant. Its original angry red color has faded to blend with my flesh. Only its bottom two inches remain darker pink and lifted in a keloid, an overgrowth of scar tissues. Almost invisible, now, are the stitch marks, while the Hemovac scars remain as puffy permanent souvenirs.

My prosthesis continues to be an irritation mentally and physically. How I hate it! It is heavy. Even separated from my chest by a cotton bra pocket, the plastic glob burns and stings my tender chest. This is a misery which I minimize by wearing a cotton undershirt beneath my bra, a solution that will be impractical when summer arrives in the southwest. Meanwhile, my body is somewhat pudgy—a fair trade to put out the fire in my chest.

For the first time in my life, I am nagged by a small spine-area ache in my upper back. Is this from not wearing the prosthesis? Or is it *from* wearing it? I really can't judge because I am so inconsistent in its use.

Breast reconstruction would eliminate the need for a prosthesis. No wonder so many women opt for reconstruction!

However this surgery is not on my agenda. Phooey to hospitals. Elective surgery is not for me; no, not even a face lift.

Except for the major change of transferring my church membership, The Big M has made surprisingly little impact on

the nitty and gritty of my life. Oh, I do try to abide by the
"Special Health Care Precautions for the Post Mastectomy
Woman," which came, via Encore, from the M. D. Anderson
Hospital and Tumor Institute in Houston. So now I carry my
purse and suitcase in my left hand, when I remember. I wear
my wristwatch and jewelry on my left arm, when I remember.
I avoid poking at cuticles and hangnails, when I remember. I
wear heavy gloves when working in the yard, when I remember. I sew with a thimble, when I remember. I don't lift heavy
objects or move furniture unassisted.

What I do, with admirable memory, is apply a lotion with
lanolin after a bath, avoid sunburn, prohibit the taking of
blood pressure and blood samples from my right arm, and ban
injections in my right arm. What I never do, and should, is
wear a loose-fitting rubber glove when my hands are in
detergent. Also, I should use insect repellent to avoid bites.

All these precautions protect my arm from uncomfortable
swelling.

I have quit Encore. Admirable as the program is, it casts
an emotional weight on me, probably because my mind is
cancer-saturated. Once this diary is done, perhaps I will be
able to return to Encore.

To me, Bosom Buddies remains an upbeat and supportive
group. What a lucky year we have experienced! Those of us on
chemotherapy are doing well. Wigs are discarded as hair
grows back. Not one of us has suffered a recurrence.

Can our luck hold? We are close friends now, and another's setback will be ours, too. We assure each other that we
can handle whatever might come.

I pray we won't be tested.

My young friend who had cancer of a salivary gland is
employed now as a nurse, his checkups perfect.

All is not flawless, of course. I wish doctors would supply
cancer-threatened women with printed pros and cons regarding mastectomy and its alternatives. In a state of shock, one
can't retain all that the doctor explains. And sure as God

makes little green apples, the new mastectomee will encounter
arguments that amputation is an unnecessarily harsh treatment for breast cancer.

Hopefully the time will come when no woman with cancer
will lose her breast. Oh, that glorious future! Alas, the date is
not here yet.

There is much available to read. This past year I have
built my knowledge of my disease and its treatment until I see
a total picture. I acted correctly, I believe, in my gamble for
continued life.

I am happy and content; blue moments come to me only
fleetingly. Louis and I live our lives as before, very intimate,
the two of us. Nothing is changed between us.

It is time now to look ahead, to live my second year after
mastectomy.

And then my third.

And then many more.

DECEMBER 1979–
NOVEMBER 1980

DECEMBER 1979

Thirteen Months After Surgery

In the weeks following my mastectomy, I considered myself a sitting duck for more cancer. If malignant cells were out to get me, there was nothing I could do to protect myself. I could only wait, then battle new cancer when it became visible.

How wrong I was!

Currently the press is providing me with concrete instructions on how to reduce my risk of cancer.

Eat less, I am told.

Eat a balanced, low-fat, high-fiber diet.

Drink alcohol only in moderate amounts.

These suggestions from the National Cancer Institute sound familiar, do they not? Obese and coronary patients know them well. How lucky that the same sane dietary rules pertain to us all!

Now if only I can put these good ideas into practice! I am to emphasize fruits, vegetables, bread, and fiber cereals, and limit dairy fats and meat. While research remains short of being Gospel, the articles I read indicate that there is a link between dairy fats, meat, and cancer, particularly cancer of the breast and colon.

Yes, National Cancer Institute, I'm listening! I'm listening! I've got to remember your advice at parties, and shun a third drink. Two highballs, three four-ounce glasses of wine, or four glasses of beer are suspected to be the daily upper limits, alas. Alcohol may act to promote cancer in cooperation with another substance.

It has been known for years that smoking vastly increases the risk of throat area and lung cancer. Current publicity introduces the idea that smoking depresses the body's immune system. For cancer patients on chemotherapy, this suggests that the effects of the drugs might be negated by smoking. It is not yet time to say that smoking depresses the body's immune system enough to give new cancers a comfortable foothold. But it might. Why chance it?

The suggestion that vitamin C is an anti-cancer agent is publicized at intervals by scientists in various countries, but it is neither endorsed nor denied by my own doctors. I take two five-hundred mg eight-hour, timed-release capsules of vitamin C daily, medicating myself. Please don't do as I do, without checking with your doctor.

I reread this segment of my diary and realize that the pattern for healthy living is not difficult. All I must do is break a few lifetime, ingrained habits.

Yep, that's all.

Thursday, December 20

My menstrual period ended one week ago and my left breast has lost its tenderness, so this is the date for BSE, breast self-examination. When the long-desired time arrives that I no longer menstruate, I will do BSE on the first day of each month.

This occasion is not a high spot of my month. Although I know that this particular fifteen minutes might once again save my life, I always perform the needed routine reluctantly, feeling narcissistic. I suspect other women react the same way and therefore hasten the procedure, or omit it.

Certainly the haphazard poking I did before my mastectomy bears no resemblance to the proper method of BSE.

I was just lucky, back in July 1978, when I first discovered my pencil stub of a growth.

Now I wait until I am alone, no interruptions expected. I divide my BSE into three separate operations: at the mirror, in the tub or shower, lying down.

My cheeks blush pink when I stand nude at the mirror, squinting critically at my Cyclops of a chest. What I am hunting is any change from the way my breast looked the month before. Is the nipple pointing differently? Does it look as if it is beginning to turn itself outside-in? Have I sensed a tingling or drawing sensation in the nipple? Is there a sore on the nipple or its areola?

I stand facing the mirror for a front-view survey, attempting to let my arms relax at my sides. A lamp shines from the side. After I have finished inspecting the front view, I turn slowly, one side to the other, letting the light cast its shadows across my chest. Sometimes it is a difference in lighting and angle that reveals a flaw.

I am comparing my breast—and my flat right side—against what I saw a month earlier. Are there any new bulges, moles, distortions, dimples, dents? Is my skin puckered? Is the contour the same? Has the breast increased or decreased in size since last month? Is there a patch of "orange peel skin"—skin that is raised, shiny, firm, and marked with deep, enlarged pores? Are there areas of redness that might signal a cancer-fighting increase in blood supply? Are blood vessels unexplainably prominent?

Change is my operative word. Should the slightest difference emerge, I will race to a doctor. "Wait and watch" regarding cancer is not in my lexicon.

After I pivot with relaxed arms, I lift my arms and lock my hands behind my head, pulling my elbows back. This puts a stretch across my chest. In this pose, I repeat the entire inspection, front view and pivoting.

And then I do it all again, with my hands pressing downward on my hips.

And then I do it all again, with my hands pushed tightly together in front of my forehead.

And then I do it all again, leaning forward from my waist so that my breast points straight down toward the floor. This is the BSE position some doctors claim is the most telling of all.

What I am doing, of course, is hunting for any tumor that

might be attached to the skin, to the chest wall, or to the ligaments within the breast. These are the villain tumors. By changing the position of my arms, I am moving skin and muscle and ligaments, and I am viewing my breast from various angles, by various lights.

Should a tumor be attached to skin or chest wall or ligaments, it will prohibit its "host" from moving in a normal way. It will exert a tug of some sort and thereby create a dimple, bulge, or other clue to cancer.

If only we women would clue hunt once a month, we would cut breast cancer deaths in half, according to some medical prophets.

I am still at the mirror, and one mirror-front chore remains. Gently, gently I squeeze my nipple, watching for secretions. Secretions are common and often harmless; again, I am hunting for a symptom which is *different*.

The possibility of secretions also is the reason that I inspect my brassiere nightly; if there should be a discharge or bleeding from the nipple, a doctor must be informed.

Well, I have gazed at my naked reflection in the mirror about as long as I can tolerate, and now I am ready for a soothing tub bath or an invigorating shower, depending on my mood. Usually I opt for the tub.

I soap my chest generously. The slippery lather is supposed to aid my sense of touch. Sitting tall, I put my left hand on the back of my head. With my right hand I check my left breast—my only breast!—for lumps. Were I one of those fortunate women blessed with impressive quantities of breast flesh, I would support my left breast with my left hand during the examination.

Having done all the preliminary work, I'm not about to short-change myself now. I examine my entire chest area from armpit to armpit, from collarbones to an inch below the bottom bulge of breast flesh. Month to month I alternate the "concentric circle method" and the "clock method," just in case I should be skipping an area accidently. Using the concentric circle method, I imagine four ever-larger rings surrounding my nipple like a bull's-eye target. Bigger breasted women need more rings. Each ring will be an examination unit.

My skin, my index finger, and my middle finger move as one, pressing in circles over the breast tissue that lies beneath the skin. My fingers are flat; fingertips can't do this job properly. I test the entire outer ring, then move just inside it to begin another circuit.

When I reach the nipple area I sense a difference, a granular condition that is normal.

On alternate months when I use the clock method I mentally divide my breast into twelve sections, like slices of pie. I begin at twelve o'clock to test the tissue, moving in to the nipple, then reversing and aiming toward the one o'clock position, pausing there to check the armpit, testing en route to the two o'clock position, going from two in to the nipple, then from the nipple out to three o'clock, from four o'clock in to the nipple, from the nipple to five o'clock, and so on, rocking around the clock.

On occasion, tumors hide directly behind a nipple; I must not forget to check there for lumps or thickening.

What I am hunting is any oddity that is attached to the skin. Or to the chest wall. Or to ligaments. Danger is greatest *if the lump does not move.*

Such a fixed lump may seem to be attached by bands or fibers. When one pinches the skin above it, *the skin won't pull away from the lump.*

None of this did I know in November 1978. Clued in by my friends' biopsy experiences, I actually had been hunting harmless cysts, marbles that moved freely. Consequently I'd almost disregarded the ropelike, non-moving stub of pencil at the bottom of my right breast.

There had been no excuse for my stupidity. Or had there been? Never had I been taught BSE in school or by a doctor. Magazine articles were helpful in technique but muddy in defining a dangerous lump. Mine, indeed, was not a lump at all.

So much for retrospection. Now my left breast has been

examined. I switch my attentions to my right chest, my right hand behind my head, my left hand probing my right armpit and my flat right chest. I pay particular attention to the incision line where recurrences are apt to root.

At last, I am two-thirds done with this monthly chore, a process that I hate despite its obvious merit. At this point I am always ready to quit, but I go on because some breast peculiarities are evident only when a woman is reclining.

Lying on my bed, I stuff a pillow or folded towels under my left shoulder in such a way that my breast is resting on the chest wall and not flopping to either side—not that it would. Cupcakes don't flop.

Anyhow, it is time again to perform either the concentric circle or the clock method, to hunt again for lumps and thickenings. My left hand is behind my head as my right hand searches my left breast.

Were I large-breasted, I would use my left hand to steady the flesh while my right fingers explored.

Of course I check my flat right chest once again, and the right armpit.

Am I done at last? Not quite. I repeat the routine with my idle arm relaxed at my side.

Now, at last, I can continue with my day and the rest of my month, knowing that I have done all in my power to find early cancer, all that I can do at home to save my own life. Rest assured that I will flee to a doctor should I discover any new lump, thickening, dimple, or nipple discharge. These are not necessarily omens of cancer, but they are symptoms that call for the judgment of an expert.

Even now, I am not completely comfortable with my routine of BSE. Ligaments worry me because my cancer was similar to a thickened ligament. Grape-like lumps come and go. I worry a lot.

To become confident of one's BSE technique requires practice, like piano playing, like CPR, like driving a car. . . . What we aim for is familiarity with our own breasts, so that we can recognize any change. *Change* is the watchword.

JANUARY 1980

In my research, I keep encountering the word "mutilation" to describe radical mastectomy. I object!

I am not mutilated. I am merely back to basics. The right side of my chest is as it was when I was age 10, with a scar added, with a nipple subtracted.

Had the deeper, muscle-removing technique of a Halsted radical been necessary, I would feel the same. We mastectomees have traded flesh for life. We are neither freaks nor cripples.

FEBRUARY 1980

Cancer treatment centers intrigue and fascinate me—from a safe and healthy distance. Being inquisitive, I jump at an opportunity to view a videotape about Houston's M.D. Anderson Hospital and Tumor Institute. The tape is to be run locally at a meeting of One Step at a Time, the support organization for cancer patients and their families.

The group meets in a school. I enter uncertainly. After Dr. DeHaven greets me, I feel more relaxed.

Some twenty-five of us sit at a horseshoe of tables and introduce ourselves.

"I am John Green and I have cancer of the pancreas, and I have quit chemotherapy because it makes me so sick."

"We are Agnes and Arnold Treat, and our seventeen-year-old daughter has bone cancer. She is not here with us tonight because she is in the hospital."

"I am Zefra Jones, I had a mastectomy, I'm taking chemotherapy, and I'm doing fine."

Almost every speaker appends, "I am doing fine."

When it is my turn to introduce myself, I say, "I am

Dorothy Abbott and my breast cancer was caught so early that I didn't need treatment beyond surgery—and I am doing fine." My words emerge with difficulty because my throat is clogged with pity for these brave people, and I know pity is not what they seek.

Too, I feel a peculiar guilt because I escaped so easily.

The patients urge John Green to go back into treatment. "We know how you feel," they insist. They express love for the teen-ager who is suffering a set-back just now. They ask Zefra Jones about the livestock and crops on her ranch.

Obviously, they like each other a lot.

Through it all, Dr. DeHaven listens, learning. We, too, learn, from his low-key comments, from his honest replies to sincere and troubled questions.

Indeed, this organization is a "support group."

We view the film.

When the meeting ends, the secretary asks if I want my name added to her membership list, if I want postcard notification of meetings.

I hesitate. I don't find One Step at a Time depressing, as my Bosom Buddy Gloria does.

I find it inspirational.

But I feel like excess baggage. There is nothing I can contribute.

"Don't send postcards," I advise the secretary. "I'll watch the newspaper and come when I can."

I've never gone back.

MARCH 1980

Call me "Limpy."

When I arise from bed or a chair, I feel pain like the sharp thrust of a hypodermic needle deep in my left hip. The pain causes me to limp for three or four steps until my brain's message reaches my legs: Walk normally.

I am annoyed. I am much too young to be lame. My common sense tells me that this is a temporary hitch-in-mygitalong, but an occasional doubt nags at me. Has a drifting cell of cancer seeded itself in my hip?

Of course not! What a dumb idea!

I promise myself that, if the pain continues, I will consult a doctor in mid-May, when we return from vacation. Surely the pain will be ended by then.

APRIL 1980

Monday, April 7

Louis reaches into tissue paper for his birthday gift, and I watch his face carefully.

He lifts out the plaque of composition stone, peers at it, and responds properly. He roars with laughter.

I have planned ahead for this anniversary, ordering a "masterpiece" from the Metropolitan Museum of Art in New York City. It is a reproduction of an Egyptian limestone relief dating from the Ptolemaic period, 332–30 B.C.

The plaque is of the upper torso and head of an Egyptian queen. Her skull is encased in an intricate, bird-shaped helmet. Her torso boasts a rounded, youthful, firm bosom.

One bosom.

Of course it is this detail that convulses Louis.

Must I grant that the second breast is assumed hidden by the Queen's braided hair? Or that this is an ancient Egyptian technique of depicting semi-profile?

I like to believe otherwise. Ancient Egyptians, I have read, did perform breast surgery, at least on men. I like to think that this catalogue-famous queen is akin to the cyclops, the unicorn, and me.

MAY 1980

Monday, May 19

Seville, Spain

The dimly-lighted ramp with its right-angle turnings seems topless. Louis and I are climbing the 250-foot Giralda, a Moorish-built tower that looms over Seville.

I drag my feet.

"Are you all right?" Louis questions. "Do you want to turn back?"

"No!" I am determined to reach the top. For the view, of course. But more emphatically to prove that I can do it.

My hip screams all the way. By now, it is obvious that exercise will not cure it, at least not the walking-down-cobble-stone-streets kind of exercise.

No longer is the pain a mere stab; now it is more general, as though my hip were bruised.

It is not black-and-blue. I have checked. So what is gnawing at that hip?

No worry on earth is strong enough to mar the view from the top of the Giralda. Seville spreads gloriously in every direction, and beyond it, the countryside of Andalusia. We spot the bull ring, the Alcazar, magnificent Maria Luisa park, the Guadalquivir river. . . . We peer straight down at the many-spired roof of the cathedral.

In a way, I set my emotions to music. *The pain in Spain falls mainly on the hip.*

When we return home, I promise myself, I will consult an orthopedist.

JUNE 1980

Monday, June 9

The crone who guards our local orthopedist tells me there is a five-month wait for hip examination, unless I have a referral from my family doctor.

The closest thing I have to a "family doctor" is my internist, Dr. Clarkly. I phone his office and beg for a referral.

"You had better see Doctor, first," his appointments girl tells me.

Dr. Clarkly knows exactly where to poke to lift me three feet off the examining table. I yelp.

"Bursitis," he decides.

We are old friends; I forgive him his grin.

Soberly, he informs me, "The best treatment is rest."

"You mean—no tennis?" Gloom is settling fast.

My ardor for tennis is recognized by him, so he refuses to embroil himself, other than to point out, "You're the one to decide what hurts and what doesn't."

"It hurts when I rest, and it hurts when I move," I complain. I suspect that nothing will erase this pain, and to quit tennis would be an empty gesture.

"Let's see if rest is the cure," he suggests. Then he hits me with a whammy. "Because of your cancer history, we had better get that hip X-rayed."

He phones immediately for my appointment.

Wednesday, June 11

The idea that a cell of my breast cancer might have escaped, traveled, and seeded itself in the bone is not a revelation to me. I have read too much about cancer to be surprised. Actually, the possibility of metastasis is one that I have recognized and dismissed.

I have blocked it from my mind for the entire three and a half months that I have been limping. Surely nothing is wrong with me except the normal wear and tear of fifty-four years.

But since Dr. Clarkly brought it up. . . .

I can't focus my mind on a happy future; instead, I keep priming myself for the bravery that I must demonstrate, should cancer recur. Bravery is what I owe my family, my friends. . . . I guess I even owe it to my doctors.

Fear is a shadow that chills me, and I must wait my turn for X rays, for a reading of those X rays, for the radiologist's report to reach Dr. Clarkly. I know Dr. Clarkly won't stall: He is efficient and, no doubt, he guesses my turmoil.

Today, Wednesday, I know immediately from his voice on the telephone that all is well. His bad-news voice echoes in a different tone.

He tells me that the X rays don't reveal why I have pain.

There has to be a reason, I rebel silently.

Dr. Clarkly drones on, reading, ". . . nor is there any indication of metastatic malignancy."

Breath huffs from my whole body, as if it has been trapped in every cavity, not only in my lungs. I sag.

Later I check "metastasis" in the dictionary although I am confident of its meaning. Surprise, there are three meanings! The first applies to me. Pathology: *Transmission of disease from an original site to one or more sites elsewhere in the body, as in tuberculosis or cancer.*

Dr. Clarkly does not dwell on the "metastatic malignancy" business. He hurries on.

"There is one thing that bears watching. You have a bone island in your left upper leg," he tells me.

"Bone island?" It is a new phrase to me.

In the months ahead I will piece together a definition that satisfies me. Apparently the island, in the marrow of the bone, is a spot that was injured or somehow deprived of blood flow. Calcium rushed in to compensate, and now the island shows up bright white on X rays.

"Lots of people have bone islands," Dr. Clarkly assures me. "Probably this one is unrelated to your present pain. However, Dr. Pelt, the radiologist, recommends that if your pain continues, you should repeat the X rays in three months."

I have no intention of limping for three more months! Maybe I'll cut down on the tennis.

JULY 1980

Thursday, July 3

To sit at this typewriter hour after hour does nothing to soothe my aching hip.

But I can't help it, can I? I'm a writer. I've been a writer since age eleven. Habits of forty-three years are difficult to break.

Only last year I was asking myself, "Why work so hard? Who needs these words I drudge out so painfully? I had cancer: I might not live to spend my royalties.

"I should be having fun."

But writing is fun, I guess, in its terrible and punishing way. Each new month I find myself spending increased time battling illusive ideas, recalcitrant paragraphs. Consequently I'm not moving about quite so much, and my body signals its distress. Plainly, I need more exercise.

But how can I exercise when my hip puts a brake on every movement?

What causes this pain? Is it cancer?

Wednesday, July 16

Now there are three-month intervals between my post-surgery checkups. Today's appointment with Dr. DeHaven is uneventful. Even the ropelike tissue at three o'clock seems to have diminished.

Friday, July 25

I am irked with myself. Life is so precious, and here I am sleeping my hours away. I nap both morning and afternoon, and by 10 P.M. I am in bed for the night.

What is the matter with me?

I know. I crave exercise. This summer has been scorching hot, too unpleasant for walking far. And didn't Dr. Clarkly recommend that I rest my hip? It does hurt when I walk.

The sun never scorches too hotly on the tennis courts, of course, for tennis freaks like me, but I have stowed my racquet. My decision was thorny, dictated in the end by my impatience to heal the hip, once and for all.

But how I hate the fatigue brought on by inactivity! I droop. I am so dull! How can anyone endure having me around?

Confident that breaststroke is great for my recalcitrant right arm, I drag myself to the neighborhood pool where I meet a woman who tells me about a YMCA program called Aquacize, in which she is an ardent participant. Exercises are done in the water where it is easier to lift arms and legs because of the water's buoyancy. With this kind of exercise, she tells me, one doesn't pay the ordinary dues of stiff, sore muscles.

She goes on to say that Aquacize is of particular value to people with physical problems: obesity, arthritis, faulty circulation, orthopedic trouble. . . .

What a way to dignify my hip pain: orthopedic trouble!

That the Aquacize class meets three mornings a week does give me pause—I write most productively in the morning—but I am fired by the necessity to DO SOMETHING.

This very day I drive downtown to the YMCA and pay my twenty-five dollar fee for the fall session which begins August 29.

AUGUST 1980

Friday, August 8

I feel punk.

My hip hurts.

When I awaken, my right arm is numb, as if I have slept on it. It is necessary to exercise away the morning stiffness.

As the day progresses, my arm grows heavier. I brace it whenever possible on the back of a sofa, on a pillow atop a chair arm, on the ledge beneath the car window on the passenger's side, on the back of a church pew. . . .

By nightfall, an invisible band grips my arm tightly from shoulder to elbow, although the mirror shows no obvious swelling. I try to sleep on my back, with my right arm propped on a pillow.

The experience of mastectomy has aged me. My face is etched with new, deep lines. My skin is pale from its decreased exposure to sunlight. Instead of remaining easily at 115 pounds, I starve to hold at 120.

It is hot, and my prosthesis burns. How I hate it!

I sit here at my typewriter and brood because this was to have been an upbeat and inspiring diary of a mastectomy, unlike earlier books in its genre. Moreover, I feel uncomfortable and unfamiliar with this catalogue of complaints. It is not my nature to mope.

All my grievances telescope into one nutshell: as I self-examine my remaining breast, what I touch feels ominously different from last month. The rope at three o'clock has returned.

Tuesday, August 12

Dr. Clarkly says that is NOT cancer at three o'clock. He says everything about my left breast seems very natural and normal to him.

I feel neither elation nor surprise. What has happened to my emotions since November 16, 1978? Have I built a wall so insulated that it separates me from joy as well as from sorrow?

Dr. Clarkly insists that I have a new mammogram; it has been eleven months since the last. I argue as always, citing the negative reading of my mammogram the very week of surgery, citing my dense breast that X ray doesn't penetrate, citing the publicized danger of X ray in encouraging cancers.

As always, Dr. Clarkly replies that the tiny amount of X ray from a mammogram is small risk compared with missing an early cancer that mammogram might find. I can't help wondering if he is a trifle uncertain, a trifle suspicious, about that ropelike tissue at three o'clock.

So once again, reluctantly, I agree to a mammogram.

Dr. Clarkly and I continue with the routine of my annual physical examination. The chest X ray is clear, free from indication of metastasis. The blood contains what it is supposed to contain, with no flags of danger.

Twenty-one months after mastectomy, all remains well.

Monday, August 18

With no breast lump, a patient waits her turn, and it is six days after my annual physical exam before my new mammogram and appointment with Dr. Pelt, the radiologist.

Again the mammograms are taken over and over; I move, they tell me.

My recent scare with the lump in the left breast that wasn't a lump continues to haunt me, and I ask Dr. Pelt his opinion of removing the second breast for safety's sake.

He is opposed, except for good cause, but he grants, "You sure can't get breast cancer in a breast that isn't there."

I confide, "I don't intend to act on this idea."

"Good girl!" he says.

He reminds me to practice BSE. As if I could possibly

forget this lifesaving procedure! On his part, he promises to watch my future mammograms for changes.

I still question whether mammograms are of value, in my case.

Friday, August 29

There is one frightening aspect to Aquacize, which begins today. When it is over, it will be necessary to strip off my wet swimming suit in the common dressing room.

How can I peel off my suit in public? How can I expose my crazy, one-breasted chest to complete strangers?

To reach the YMCA I wear my street clothes over my swimsuit, my expensive mastectomy swimsuit with its stiff B-cups mountaining over my A-sized left bosom and my right-sided flatness. Suits with A-cups are not available. There is no point in sewing pockets into this suit; my prosthesis would drift around like a marshmallow in a cup of hot chocolate.

That prosthesis in its bra is tucked deeply into my beach-bag, along with panties and a towel.

I gravitate to the rear of the dressing room, where rows of lockers promise some shielding. There I deposit my skirt and t-shirt and shoes. When I slam my locker door, it resounds with a metallic echo of finality that tells me: Your bridges are burned. March forward.

I march.

The water is soothingly warm. Nobody is swimming. All the ladies are jogging across the pool, the water resistance causing them to bounce as they progress, and I think wildly of the India rubber ball in *A Child's Garden of Verses*.

Many of the ladies are fleshy, in extreme contrast to our teacher, who is lean and willowy in her skin-tight nylon tank suit.

We stretch.

We kick.

We breathe deeply.

I see similarities to yoga, but these exercises are easier, thanks to the support of the water. My hip is hurting, but I can bear it.

The class ends, and I ponder driving home in my wet suit. Or I could dart into a toilet enclosure to dress.

But that wouldn't cure this self-consciousness of mine. It is essential that I behave like everybody else because I *am* like everybody else.

I'll see this through, I decide. My lower lip is thrust forward, I know.

After a shower with my suit on, I find there is only one other person in my secluded nest of lockers, a girl with red-gold curls piled high on her head. She is seven months pregnant.

We talk. I maneuver my towel constantly between us, and I am suddenly aware that this is not through shame or modesty. What I am doing is protecting this youngster from a female fact-of-life. In her pregnancy, she is already saturated in what it means to be a woman. Why should she be forced to handle more?

SEPTEMBER 1980

Wednesday, September 17

When one meets three mornings a week with the same people, for the same purpose, walls begin crumbling. A camaraderie grows.

My wall is my towel, and gradually I become able to peel off my suit in the shower, to parade around wrapped in a towel, actually to expose my front while I wipe my back and legs.

Nobody stares at me.

Nor do they glance and cringe and turn away.

We women are in this together, after all.

My Bosom Buddy Loretta is home from vacation and doing Aquacize. One morning after class I ask her to zip my zipper.

She obliges, but she says, loudly, "You should do this yourself. It's good for your arm, to stretch it."

"I know," I agree, "but I couldn't manage this zipper even before my silly surgery." My voice matches hers in loudness. Might a listener realize this public announcement is a milestone for me?

In this once-dreaded dressing room, I examine Loretta's chest with its eighteen-year-old scars from her double radical mastectomy. Her breastbone forms a shelf over a much-indented flat chest.

In contrast, the right side of my chest drops straight down from my breastbone exactly as it did before puberty. This is the difference between Loretta's Halsted radical and my "modified" radical. Her pectoral muscles are gone and mine are not.

In the sixteen years between her operation and mine, the modified radical mastectomy, as the way to deal with outer quadrant tumors, has become the preferred technique by many surgeons but not all. Some still insist upon doing the operation developed by Dr. William S. Halsted in the late 1800's, despite nearly identical survival rates. I abhor the word "mutilation" when linked with mastectomy, and I reject it totally, but I am grateful that my chest is not like Loretta's.

Sunday, September 21

This morning I read, once again, a newspaper report indicating that, possibly, the elimination of caffeine from one's diet will diminish fibrocystic breast disease. It is a claim that I have been encountering since my surgery, when I became poignantly alert to such articles.

As women age, fibrocystic breast disorder is common. What happens is that the woman's body creates an excess amount of fibrous tissue. This extra, ropelike tissue tends to obstruct the woman's mammary ducts, creating a dam behind which fluids accumulate. The trapped fluids stretch the ducts in about the same way air stretches a balloon, and the resultant round, firm, smooth masses are called cysts. Such cysts vary in size during a menstrual cycle and are tender to pressure. One nurses' dictionary defines the condition as "small nodules like buckshot," and its accompanying pain as "the shooting type."

Contents of such cysts can be aspirated by needle in a doctor's office.

So this morning I sit at the breakfast table with two complete Sunday newspapers mounding around me, and I realize, *This is something I can do.* Part of my frustration in being a cured cancer patient has been my inability *to do something* to ward off recurrence. It is such a tied-hands feeling!

In the past when I questioned Dr. Clarkly about giving up coffee, he said, "You know as much about it as I do. The medical journals don't reveal any information you haven't read in the newspaper. It seems some women benefit. The evidence is still too skimpy to make a judgment.

"By-the-way," he said to me, frowning, "how much coffee do you drink?"

Years ago when I was writing seriously, I kept coffee on my desk all morning. Recently, I have been limiting myself to two and a half cups, all at breakfast.

I love coffee! I love it! Can I exist without it? Suddenly I want to try. Doesn't it make sense that if a woman rids herself of benign lumps a cancer will stand free and clear? With the fibrocystic "bunches of grapes" absent, shouldn't a malignancy be more obvious? If I'm to have cancer again, I want it discovered fast.

The newspaper article warns that I must give up tea, too,

and chocolate, and soft drinks, and certain over-the-counter drugs including Anacin, Excedrin, Dristan, Midol, No Doz, and Vanquish.

Sadly, I stare into my mug with its super-strong, aromatic nectar, brewed the way I love it. Is this beverage stronger than my self-discipline?

Without a farewell sip, I pour the heavenly stuff down the sink.

I'm off coffee, cold turkey.

Thursday, September 25

To my astonishment, I'm suffering no withdrawal symptoms. My taste buds aren't clamoring for caffeine. My nerves aren't jumping. My head isn't aching.

For breakfast I drink boiling water poured over a slice of lemon. At least it's hot.

Monday, September 29

My hip continues to hurt, and I worry that I am causing damage with Aquacize. Dutifully, I return to the radiologist for repeat X rays of my left hip.

Nothing has changed since the June X rays. The bone island remains the same. There is no sign of malignancy.

"Why do I hurt?" I wail.

"I only know about the bones," Dr. Pelt tells me, "and the bones aren't causing your pain. We'll X-ray again in six months if the pain continues."

Six more months? Ridiculous! I want the answers now.

Tuesday, September 30

When Dr. Clarkly phones with the X-ray results, which I already know, I insist on his getting me a prompt appointment with Dr. Breen, the orthopedist. I crave exercise—but I must exercise without damaging myself permanently.

I'm still uncertain about the effect of Aquacize on my hip. I resent my fruitless lay-off from tennis. Without tennis I am droopy and fatigued, and separated from friends. I'm getting mighty annoyed with medical run-around.

Can no doctor cure my hip pain?

OCTOBER 1980

Wednesday, October 8

Can no doctor cure my hip pain?

Apparently not.

Dr. Breen, a friend of long standing, grins and then reminds me, "Both of us are getting older."

As I follow him down the hall to view my newly-shot back X rays, we both are limping.

My lower back is a mess. Spurs on the bone. Spaces between the vertebrae, some too large and some too small. Arthritis.

The source of my hip pain is in my lower back, Dr. Breen tells me. There is no sign of cancer.

There is no sign of cancer. Once more I hear the cheering words. Pain is no big deal when its source isn't lethal.

Dr. Breen applauds my Aquacize (what a relief!) but he emphasizes that I must do nothing, absolutely nothing, that creates pain. Stop short of pain, he stresses. The same warning applies to tennis and even to walking.

Days of joy and sunshine, I can play tennis!

For the sake of my back, he tells me, I am never to grow obese. For the sake of my marriage, I tell him, I am never to grow obese.

He asks how diligent I have been with the exercises he assigned to me eighteen years ago.

Eighteen years ago!

"I did them faithfully, more or less," I remember, "until the mastectomy, and then about all I could manage was the arm exercises."

He makes it clear that my failure to stretch my back is the cause of the current distress.

Without the cancer, there would have been no mastectomy. Without the mastectomy, I would have exercised. Therefore, cancer caused my hip pain, after all.

My logic is good, I suppose, but my excuses are faulty. Of course I could have exercised my back as well as my recalcitrant arm, if only I'd set my mind to it.

Tuesday, October 21

As a guest at a large luncheon buffet, I nurse my wine and I mingle. Over and over a friend asks, "Whatever happened to Bosom Buddies? When will we all meet again?"

"I'll phone the list soon," I promise.

I count. At least seven of my Bosom Buddies are at this party. By this year's statistics, one woman in eleven will face breast cancer sometime in her life. We eight mastectomees are about in the right proportion here in this cheerful, milling crowd.

In a moment when I am uninvolved in conversation, I gaze critically at these friends who have shared my medical experience. Pride pounds at me. Don't we all look stunning?

We are standing tall.

We are wearing beautiful clothes, not too tight across the chest.

We are laughing and enjoying ourselves.

We are the same as everybody else.

Friday, October 31

I feel marvelous!

This has been a splendid week, a splendid month. The tight-squeezing band on my right upper arm has eased remarkably. The entire arm seems to weigh less, to tire more slowly.

Meanwhile the twinges in my hip are fewer and milder. I have quit limping.

The overwhelming fatigue that caused me to sleep away precious hours of my life, and impeded my waking hours, has lost its grip on me. Oh, yes, I feel great. I am making progress with a capital "P."

My writing is moving forward. Is this because I am feeling so well, or am I feeling well because my writing flows?

Has my banning of caffeine boosted my energy?

How much of my resumed good health and spirits should I credit to the passage of time, and how much to exercise? Most to exercise, I would venture. Both Aquacize and the "dry land" stretches for my back contribute to my well-being. But a single set of tennis still cripples me.

I feel good about myself because I have learned certain facts about my body that I didn't know before. I have a growing faith in my body's anti-cancer defenses. No longer am I fearful that any cancer cell that might have escaped the breast, before or during mastectomy, will ultimately colonize in bone, liver, wherever. . . . By reading, I have learned that lymph nodes throughout the body—not only in the axilla—are strainers to trap wayward cells, and that additional protection comes from other body mechanisms that are capable of killing villain invaders.

All this I have learned from reading. Why, oh why didn't one of my doctors ease my mind by pointing out these very facts? Perhaps they credited me with more wisdom and more knowledge than I possessed.

I like my chest; really I do. It amuses me, and it amuses my husband. We are unique: the cyclops, the unicorn, and I.

NOVEMBER 1980

Friday, November 7

I am procrastinating. I am postponing. Oh, why am I so reluctant to make that one hundred-mile trip to shop for new mastectomy brassieres and possibly a new prosthesis?

Alas, the elastic inserts in my original mastectomy bras have lost their resiliency. And my second prosthesis, the only one I have kept, has never been quite right. It is teardrop-shaped and I wear its tail either upright or toward my armpit, depending on the design of a bra's cup. Either way, I am left with a hollow in the uncovered area.

What I need is a prosthesis with extensions both upward and sideward, a prosthesis generally triangle-shaped. Above all, it must be comfortable.

Mastectomy brassieres with pockets for prostheses now cost about twenty dollars, and prices are skyrocketing. The average prosthesis is priced well over a hundred dollars. Some I have investigated are 250 dollars.

What is the dollar value of the silicone and other ingredients of a prosthesis? Why should a mastectomy bra cost double or triple what an ordinary bra costs? Do the economics of volume make this giant difference? Or are manufacturers and merchants gouging a trapped clientele?

Anyhow, I hang back. I suspect that I'll spend a lot of money and energy and time, only to trade one set of problems for another.

Sunday, November 16

Two Years After Surgery

Today marks the two-year anniversary of my mastectomy. It is a meaningful date because during these first two years a woman is at her greatest risk of recurrence or metastasis. My next big milestone is five years, then ten. Should I survive ten years with no more cancer, I will be considered cured.

I intend to live on. Truly I yearn to greet the year 2000.

In my greediness, I thank God fervently for the fifty-four years He already has given me, and for the years ahead. Today I am feeling sentimental and deeply grateful toward my doctors, the whole bushel of them.

I apologize to them for my fretting, for the times when I was like the boy in the legend who cried "Wolf!" No doubt future years will bring more aching bones, more breast lumps, more cancer-suggestive symptoms. It will be my responsibility to seek medical consultation. As a one-time cancer patient, I must not self-diagnose and write off my body's warnings as mere symptoms of aging. If I cry "Wolf!" ten times, and on the tenth occasion uncover an early cancer, there need be no apologies for the nine false alarms.

I am looking into the future with confidence, soothed by the fact that the battle against cancer is proceeding rapidly. Within my lifetime I have watched chemotherapy develop from being a last resort effort, when nothing else was left to offer, to a therapeutic form of treatment designed to prevent recurrence. And plans for the future of chemotherapy are startling: faster cures, easier cures, perhaps even prevention.

Consider the research devoted to "chemoprevention," the use of anti-cancer compounds to deter carcinogens from reaching vulnerable targets in the body or from gaining a foothold in these particular targets. The idea behind chemoprevention is to hasten the body's own metabolism and thus increase its natural ability to fight.

The long-term goals of cancer researchers deal both with prevention and treatment. They hunt a safe vaccine for prevention. They seek a way to strengthen the patient's own immune system, as a part of treatment.

Detection methods for breast cancer are bound to improve. Already being tested is a thin, pliable material to be tucked inside a brassiere for ten to fifteen minutes once a month. This material changes color according to temperature differences in the breast tissue. A cancer registers warmer because it demands a greater blood supply than normal cells.

Such breakthroughs are bound to speed the initial discovery of a woman's cancer. With early detection comes cure.

Today's mastectomee, at her request and with her surgeon's approval, can be visited by a Reach to Recovery volunteer and supplied with helpful pamphlets: information for her teen-aged children, information for her husband, instructions for exercise. . . . She even receives a gift packet of immediately useful items, including a soft prosthesis.

The American Cancer Society, with offices in most cities, also is a source of help, both practical (bandages, wheelchairs) and informational.

I reflect on the sunny aspect of things to come as I celebrate this, the second anniversary of my mastectomy.

But I am not completely home free. My two-year checkup is scheduled for next week.

Monday, November 24

I awaken at 5:30 A.M. and cannot fall back to sleep. My mind is hostage to the fact that this afternoon I go to Dr. DeHaven for my two-year-post-surgery checkup. What will he decide, now that the "rope" has returned to its old three o'clock position in my left breast? Alas, I know that ten per cent of women with cancer in one breast later develop cancer in the other breast. Am I to be one of the ten per cent?

My uptightness remains with me through Aquacize, through the running of my errands. Mastectomy isn't difficult but oh, dear Lord, I don't want to do it over again. At least, not quite yet.

When I reach the surgeon's examining room I am armed with a list of questions, some pertaining to my own medical experience and some double-checkings for the accuracy of this diary. As I wait for him, I don't even glance at the antique, medical doodads in the cubbyholes of his wall-mounted printer' tray. After two years of frequent appointments, I know them well.

Dr. DeHaven enters, and there is still a little of that 15-year-old kid in his step, despite the gray in his hair.

I clutch my open-down-the-front paper jacket which already has ripped beyond modesty, and I ask, "Do you want to answer my questions first or do you want to examine me first?"

"Questions first."

Another postponement in coping with that rope at three o'clock!

With a deep breath, I plunge in. "Here I am almost fifty-five years old and still menstruating regularly," I complain. "Isn't this encouraging cancer? Why wasn't an estrogen-binding study done on my cancer after the mastectomy?"

He pages through my surgical report and says, "It was done. Your cancer had a borderline dependence on estrogen. We would not have considered an oophorectomy unless you had a recurrence." From reading and my chats with Bosom Buddies, I knew that an oophorectomy was the surgical removal of one or both ovaries, the purpose being to stop the ovaries' production of cancer-feeding hormones.

"If I had known about that estrogen-binding study," I say tartly, "I might have worried less." Memories rush back, of Bosom Buddies griping that their doctors didn't detail for them the specifics of their cases, withholding facts out of kindness, perhaps, or for lack of time. *Or because a male doctor misjudged a woman's intelligence?*

For a person like me, who reads for information, the total picture is imperative. Gaps in knowledge create worry. It wasn't enough for me to know that I wasn't receiving certain common treatments; I needed to know WHY. Obviously I didn't phrase my questions properly because Dr. DeHaven always seemed to answer everything I asked.

This afternoon Dr. DeHaven goes on to explain that other factors enter into the decision for an oophorectomy including the size of the tumor and how long it has been rooted in the breast.

We discuss the new CAT (computerized axial tomography) scanner that, with more accuracy and less radiation dosage than with mammogram, screens women with high risk of breast cancer (me!) or whose diagnosis by current methods is uncertain (me, again). It is particularly effective for women with dense breasts (me).

"This is what I'm going to have, the next time," I declare. "Even if I have to go to the University of Kansas Medical Center or to the Mayo Clinic." The new machines were available only in these two locations in 1979, when women's magazines reported their development. This breast scanner is different from those CAT scanners which examine the head or the whole body.

Somehow our conversation drifts to the fact that breast cancer in men is much more aggressive than in women, and that a man's breast tumor spreads earlier. Recurrences happen discouragingly quickly. Therefore all men with breast cancer are treated with both radiation and chemotherapy.

In the past two years, Dr. DeHaven has performed mastectomies on four men. Nationally, the rate for male breast cancer is about one per cent of total cases.

The men have one advantage, I reflect. They don't have to wear a heavy, bulky, uncomfortable prosthesis.

It is time for my examination. Dr. DeHaven explores my chest, my armpits, my liver, and who-knows-what-else.

"What's that rope at three o'clock?" I ask, trembling. "It's awfully much like that cancer I had in my right breast."

"No, it isn't," he insists. "See, I can move it around. It's not attached to anything—the other one was attached."

It's not attached to anything. What beautiful words! Why hadn't my own fingers discovered this vital, soothing fact? The answer is clear: I still am clumsy and ineffective at BSE, breast self-examination.

For safety sake, and to provide comparison records for the future, Dr. DeHaven prescribes a bone scan, my first, and some blood work to check the function of my liver.

I pass all tests with flying colors. There is no cancer anywhere. If I felt any better, I would be walking on air.

Musings

Two years are past! I am alive! And I feel wonderful.

Is it too simplistic to believe that certain exercises and no caffeine have made this difference?

The ache in my upper back, troublesome a year ago, is gone. My hip remains quiet *when I don't play tennis.* What anguish this simple fact causes me! It's not fair that while mastectomy can't keep me off the courts, old bones can.

I look older. The lines in my face etch deeper. My skin is pale from my avoiding the sun, for even that sun I love and cherish is a cancer-causing agent. Now my hair is streaked with gray from time to time because I color it infrequently; hair dyes once contained suspected carcinogens, and although manufacturers have changed formulations, I remain slightly gun-shy.

Diet's suspected link with cancer remains very much on my mind. Now I cook red meat one day, chicken the next, fish the next, and we actually enjoy this rotation. In the past we consumed entirely too much beef.

And now, alas, I limit my own portions. No more "pigging it up."

There are other changes. No longer do I dread shaving under my arms. I can look back with amusement to the day when Louis laboriously trimmed my armpit with manicure scissors so that Dr. DeHaven wouldn't know I had disobeyed his orders. I just couldn't take a razor to that feelingless flesh! Now reawakened nerves guide my razor.

Too, now I can feel the bite of fingernails when I stratch my right shoulder and upper back. But neither armpit nor shoulder nor back feels quite as it did before mastectomy. Maybe next year. . . .

The healing of my chest is complete, the incision flesh-colored except for its bottom two inches of pink keloid. Perhaps this advanced healing has contributed to the comfort of my prosthesis which I wear, now, most of the time. I don't like it, but I no longer hate it. Breast reconstruction still doesn't entice me. For that matter, neither does a face lift. Maybe I'm going to delight in growing old, considering its alternative.

Meanwhile, I'm forced to keep moving and stretching because when I don't, an invisible band squeezes my upper arm, and my entire arm grows heavy and fatigued. Swelling never has been obvious, but still I find comfort in bracing my arm shoulder-high whenever possible, to encourage the drainage of fluids from that arm, drainage which had been a function of lymph nodes now gone.

My cancer-connected social life has diminished. Encore has ended for lack of participants. I cannot begin volunteer visiting with Reach to Recovery until I am two years post-op—which is right now, hurrah. Bosom Buddies languishes for lack of a volunteer to make restaurant reservations and to telephone the membership list. I'm going to do it, truly I am, the day I mail this manuscript to the publisher.

All of us Bosom Buddies continue to thrive, with nary a recurrence among us, thank God. My young friend who had cancer of the salivary gland thrives, too.

We all are advocates of the power of positive emotions. We laugh and love and fill each hour to the brim. Negative emotions, we know, might jolt our own body defenses out of whack.

I, for one, need my body working for me, not against me. Optimism is a great medicine.

As I did one year ago, I can again report that mastectomy has made surprisingly little impact on the nitty and gritty of my life. I am happy and content and busy. Louis and I live our lives as before, very intimate. Nothing is changed between us. Mastectomy isn't so bad.

CASE HISTORIES

INTRODUCTION TO CASE HISTORIES

My diary of a mastectomy is typical in that it is atypical, for no two women recover from breast surgery in exactly the same way. Some bodies heal rapidly, some mend slowly. Some arms regain full motion and never swell, others require continuing exercise and the wearing of elastic sleeves.

In the pages that follow, I relate the stories of fourteen women who have experienced breast surgery. Without question, a mastectomy is a major jolt in a woman's life, a time for introspection and evaluation. So indelible are certain patient-doctor dialogues that years later a woman can quote them word for word.

These women ranged in age from twenty-three to seventy-nine when, for the first time, they became aware of a breast irregularity. The first two underwent mastectomies in 1945, the last in 1980. Their economic backgrounds vary. They are Jewish, Protestant, and Roman Catholic.

Not by the longest stretch of the imagination could any of these women be termed "Pollyanna," yet their common response to cancer is free of anger and blame.

You will see.

1945

MARY BETH

In 1945, forty years old and with children at home, Mary Beth lost her breast to cancer. So secret was her hospitalization and recuperation that not even her closest friends were aware of her "ordeal."

"Ordeal" was a common tag for mastectomy in those days. "Nice" people didn't publicize a "personal tragedy." Concealment protected the "victim" and her associates.

Mary Beth endeavored to protect her adolescent children by never, never mentioning her surgery. Her daughters did not learn, from her, that their own risk of breast cancer was increased by hereditary factors. Breast self examination never was discussed.

Not only did Mary Beth's silence reflect her era, but it reflected her family's abhorrence of medical matters aired in public. It was the depth of bad taste, they believed, to mention symptoms, bodily flaws, or ills in social conversation. Certainly a proper lady would not discuss her breast.

Mary Beth remains in excellent health, watching grandchildren grow to adulthood. With her husband she travels and plays golf and leads an active social life, enjoying his retirement.

She successfully guards her secret. It is only by a fluke that I discovered it.

She doesn't know I know.

1945

VERA

Mary Beth's handling of her mastectomy was in complete contrast to the experience of Vera, who also lost a breast to cancer in 1945.

At the time of surgery, Vera was seventy-nine years old. To recuperate, she would live with her daughter, my friend Nona.

Nona openly discussed what was happening to her mother, in preparing for her arrival.

No sooner had Vera taken up residence in our city when certain of Nona's friends rushed to Vera's side to reveal, "I had this same surgery years ago."

Nona marvels, "In every case I was absolutely flabbergasted. I'd had not a glimmer of a hint that the friend had undergone mastectomy. The operation still was in the hush-hush category—except for a wonderful woman-to-woman camaraderie, a yearning to cheer and encourage each other.

"It wasn't a club of handholders," Nona reflects. "It was just pilgrimages by individual women with love in their hearts."

The year 1945 had not been kind to Vera. Her husband had been dying of leukemia when she noticed a lump on her breast. Frightened, she appealed to Nona for help.

Nona arrived in Kansas to find her father critically ill. Attention to Vera's lump was postponed until after his death and funeral.

Then doctors gave Vera conflicting advice. One, in Vera's home town, suggested, "Wait." Nona's own doctor shrugged off the symptom. "Aw, at your age, Vera, let's not get so worked up."

But one doctor whose specialty was in another field suggested, "Go to the Mayo Clinic in Rochester, Minnesota. As far as I know, that is the only place where there are facilities to test for cancer while the patient remains under sedation. The biopsy and the mastectomy, if necessary, can be accomplished in a single trip to the operating room."

This would save Vera the dangers of a second anesthetic and the trauma of waiting for mastectomy.

A surgeon at Mayo's was recommended.

Consulted by telephone, the surgeon said, "If you don't mind coming at Christmas, come right away."

"But it's snowing," Vera protested.

"You don't have to travel in a covered wagon," the doctor pointed out, somewhat sourly.

The day after Christmas, Vera underwent surgery. Not only was her lump a cancer, but her lymph nodes were involved.

X ray following mastectomy was the treatment of the time. As she healed, Vera moved from the hospital to a Rochester hotel to await February and her first X-ray sessions.

There was an interlude, and then more X rays.

After these initial doses, the X-ray treatment was repeated at the Mayo Clinic twice a year for four or five years, until Vera was informed, "You have passed the critical stage. There is no reason to continue treatment."

Such good news was not anticipated by Vera when she first went to live with Nona. She was suffering a triple blow: the death of her husband, the loss of her breast with its accompanying reality of cancer, and the closing of her beloved, long-time home. Her depression was understandable.

But then Nona's mastectomee friends rallied to Vera's side. Little by little, Vera's strength returned. Her arm was "tired" but never swollen.

When the housing shortages that followed World War II eased, Vera moved back to Kansas, to an apartment of her own. She remained independent almost to the end of her life.

Cancer never recurred in any form. Fourteen years after her mastectomy, Vera died.

She was ninety-three.

1952

WANDA

At age twenty-three and newly married to a marine on active duty, Wanda was soaping herself in the shower when her fingers drifted over an oddity in her left breast. Again and again her fingers returned to explore the puzzling spot.

She emerged from the shower in a daze. "Walt, honey, take a look at this," she said.

He looked, then announced, "We're going to the naval hospital."

"No, we're not. We're going to Temple," she argued. It was the Jewish New Year.

"We're going to the hospital," he repeated, with such firmness that she knew she had married a stubborn man.

Within an hour after Wanda's accidental discovery of the lump, a doctor was examining her. His decision was that because Wanda was so young, her problem must be a clogged mammary gland or something of that nature. She was instructed to go through a complete one-month cycle with weekly visits to the doctor.

All month, the lumps grew and multiplied.

A biopsy was scheduled for a Friday. Wanda entered the hospital on Thursday. It was then that the doctors decided, on the evidence of the rapidly increasing mass, that Wanda probably had cancer and mastectomy was needed.

But the hospital's surgery schedule was heavy that Friday. A biopsy could have been crammed in, but the lengthy process of mastectomy was impossible.

Wanda was told, "Go home and have a nice weekend with your husband."

Have a nice weekend with your husband.

Wanda and her bridegroom spent the days in solitude, comforting each other. They were terrified, floundering, acutely aware of their youth and inexperience.

They chose to endure the emotional crisis alone, not reaching to friends for help, not telephoning their parents.

Wanda's surgery on Monday was predicted to last two and a half hours. What a surprise when in half an hour, Walt was told, "She has no malignancy after all. She will be down from the operating room shortly."

What a perplexing but jubilant change of signals!

Even before Walt's heartbeat resumed its normal pace, he was approached by a hall-strolling, recuperating patient, the wife of a marine general. "I overheard," she said simply. "Now this is what we're going to do. I will take turns with you, standing beside Wanda's bed. We are going to tell her, over and over, that she has no cancer. That her breast is not gone."

This they did, on the theory that hearing is the first sense to return after unconsciousness. Wanda swam to consciousness knowing the good news.

In the elapsed years she often has recalled the support and kindness of that woman.

And why was the general's lady in the hospital? She herself had undergone a mastectomy a few days earlier.

Wanda healed rapidly, psychologically "up."

During her surgery, six large tumors had been removed. The pathologist judged them to be "mixed benign fibroma;" in other words, various kinds of cells, none of them cancerous.

While she remained on the operating table, the surgeon rearranged Wanda's remaining, distorted tissue into a normal breast shape, half the size of the untouched right breast. In time the left breast would fill with fatty tissue to approximately its normal size, she was promised.

Miraculously it did.

Wanda was told she could safely bear children, but that they must not be breast fed. If her distorted breast did produce sufficient milk, the nursing might be painful. The baby might sense something wrong and not nurse properly.

Wanda gave birth to four children.

Always she was extremely watchful of her breasts, examining them thoroughly before and after each period, less thoroughly at least once a week. Also, she counted on Walt to back up her investigations with his own serious examinations. They worked as a team, wary of danger.

Lumps did develop. At age thirty-three and again at thirty-nine, Wanda underwent biopsies.

"The biggie," as she calls it, hit her at age forty-six.

The laboratory report of that biopsy was ambiguous.

Fortunately, Wanda had a contact in New York City who submitted the results of her tests to three different hospitals, receiving a total of six opinions.

All six opinions were different.

One defined her problem as benign disease, with cancer to be expected in later years.

One emphasized the necessity for frequent mammograms, physical examinations, and self examination.

One judged that she had "carcinoma in situ," a localized cancer, without spread.

By this time Wanda was in anguish, hating her breasts, resenting her twenty-three years (exactly half of her life!) of ever-diligent, ever-fearful vigilance against cancer. Too, she was haunted by her mother's recent death, from cancer of another kind.

She admits, "I couldn't hack the mental part any more. I thought the physical part of the surgery was going to be easy, in comparison.

"But I didn't want only one breast removed. I had lost the emotional durability to continue self-examining. There were also aesthetic reasons. I didn't want to cope with problems of balance, and of matching a prosthesis to a remaining breast.

"I requested that both breasts be removed.

"Walt agreed."

The method selected was subcutaneous mastectomy, with Wanda's own breast skin and nipples preserved. In a single operation, both breasts and some representative lymph nodes were removed. Abnormal tissue showed up in both breasts. To everybody's relief, the nodes tested negative.

Wanda had no intention of returning to a hospital for any reason, least of all for reconstruction, an elective surgery. But in the healing process, nerve endings caught in scar tissue. Wanda suffered burning and tingling sensations all the time. Even her sleep was disturbed.

A remedy had to be sought.

During the original mastectomies, all tissue was stripped from the chest wall. Now a plastic surgeon stripped again, getting rid of pain-causing scar tissue. As part of the cure, he inserted silicone prostheses.

Wanda's pain has ended. Now she has well-shaped breasts, albeit silicone. After top layers fell away, her nipples regenerated. Nipple sensations are not as before, however.

Five years have passed.

Wanda continues to work, part time, at a job she loves. Never does she fret about the possibility of new cancers evolving from the breast site. But she is a realist. She knows that because she smokes, she may someday face lung cancer.

She is active physically; she swims frequently.

"My arms fatigue quickly. They aren't as strong or mobile as before the surgery—and that is my fault." Wanda believes that she doesn't exercise diligently enough.

She walks into corners, into doors, into walls because there is no feeling in her silicone "protrusions." It feels as if her body begins at her ribs. Thus, she misjudges distance.

Being a "bumper" tickles Wanda's funnybone. She is cheery. She is grateful and relieved that her breasts are gone.

And how have her medical experiences affected her family?

Walt has been her strength. "The impact is totally different when the husband is supportive," she reflects.

After her mastectomies and before her reconstruction, Wanda sometimes wore her prostheses and sometimes she didn't. Sometimes she was round and fully packed, sometimes pancake flat.

Her two sons begged, "Please, Mom, be consistent. Either wear them or don't wear them."

She obliged.

The boys never worried much about Wanda. "We know you can handle it, Mom," they praised. Their concern was for their younger sisters, entering puberty. How would the two girls handle the knowledge that their brand-new breasts—and indeed their very lives—were at risk due to the strong hereditary nature of breast cancer?

The girls, in their high-school years, steered clear of the subject. Now, as adults, they introduce breast cancer as a topic during close mother-daughter chats. "I don't have a good outlook, do I?" one asked recently, revealing her concern.

Remembering that her own first lump was found by lucky accident, Wanda is comforted by the fact her daughters regularly practice breast self-examination, BSE. They are at risk, of course. But cancer detected early is cancer that can be cured.

1954

CAROL

Carol gave birth to a daughter and a son after she lost a breast to cancer, putting her into a class almost by herself.

"Breast cancer is an older woman's disease. What you have is a cyst," said Carol's doctor, in her small West Texas town. The year was 1954. Carol was twenty-five.

Having been married three years without a pregnancy, Carol was at this time undergoing tests to discover whether her ovarian tubes were blocked. The office procedure of blowing air into the tubes, repeated several times, had been inconclusive as well as painful.

"We'll have to repeat the tests in the hospital, under sedation," the doctor decreed. "And as long as you're going to be under sedation, we might as well biopsy that breast lump that's worrying you." Previously he had prescribed medication to dissolve the "cyst."

By this time Carol had noticed a change in her lump. When first discovered, it had been the size and shape of a small hen's egg, and smooth to the touch, as if confined by a shell. After medication the outside of the lump became bumpy, as if the contents were spilling out of a broken shell.

"I feel certain this is when the cancer started to spread," she reflects. "If only the biopsy had come first! The cancer was all neatly encapsulated at the beginning, I believe."

In 1954, West Texas was not heavily populated with pathologists. Carol's tissue was sent to Amarillo for testing.

"If it's positive, they'll phone us," the doctor promised. "If it's negative, they'll send a letter."

The biopsy took place on a Thursday. Carol went home from the hospital on Friday. No telephone call Friday. None Saturday. None Sunday. Carol and her husband began to breathe easier. So did her doctor, no doubt.

On Monday Carol phoned for a doctor's appointment because her incision looked puffy.

It was late Monday afternoon when patient and doctor met in his examining room. The doctor eyed the incision.

"That's just natural serum, not infection," he judged. After a long pause, he added, "Get dressed. I want to see you in my office."

What now? Carol wondered, dressing rapidly.

She froze on the threshold of the office. Her husband was there, waiting.

Her heart stood still. *What is this?* she remembers wondering, although she already knew.

Her biopsy had tested positive.

The doctor offered a long-winded explanation for the delay. The Amarillo pathologist was away on vacation. Carol's tissue had been, of necessity, forwarded from Amarillo to Fort Worth for examination.

The phone message from the Fort Worth laboratory had reached the doctor's wife at their home late Sunday night. She took the message to him in the bathroom, where he was brushing his teeth, preparing for bed.

Upon hearing the news, he vomited.

Carol would undergo mastectomy at age twenty-five.

Carol's early morning request for an appointment had saved the doctor the sad chore of phoning her.

From a list of recommended surgeons, Carol picked one blindly because he practiced in Dallas where her parents-in-law lived. Her husband could bunk with them while she was in the hospital.

On Wednesday, Carol and her husband drove the long distance to Dallas.

On Thursday the surgeon prodded the swollen lymph nodes beneath Carol's arm. "It looks as though the cancer has spread," he noted with a frown. "We should do a radical mastectomy."

Carol entered the hospital.

The "radical" was performed on Friday.

In Dallas and elsewhere, post-surgery treatment of breast cancer was in a transition stage in 1954, X ray no longer the sole therapy, extensive use of cobalt radiation and chemotherapy yet to come. This was the era of radium treatment.

Vials of radium particles were inserted into Carol's body in two steps, the first while she was under anesthetic for the mastectomy, the second on the day after surgery.

It was during the surgery that six radium-filled vials were inserted along Carol's breastbone. Radiation emitted from the particles were to create a fence that would kill any loose malignant cells that might be on their way to her other breast.

Carol was told that the radium particles were like fine grains of sand, and that the vials were of platinum.

"I was expensive, there for a while," she jokes.

The next day six more vials of radium were inserted above Carol's collarbone, in order to block any cancer cells that might be traveling to her neck. These were shot into place with a kind of gun, causing extreme pain. No medication was given to ease the pain.

For the next twenty-four hours Carol suffered intense pain from the radium's action. Morphine was on her chart, but nobody told her she could have it. When morphine finally was administered, it took three shots within two hours to ease her suffering.

The twelve radium vials remained in place during her week of hospitalization, during which time she also underwent daily X-ray treatments.

The week ended.

Carol's surgeon removed the breastbone vials "with a gadget that popped them right out." Consequently, Carol was unprepared for the torture of the extraction of the neck-area vials, done without anesthetic. Since she had healed in that area, a scalpel was used.

"The nurse said, 'Hang onto me,' and I damn near broke her hand." Even today, Carol winces at the memory.

Her souvenir from the neck area treatment is a strawberry mark similar to a birthmark. Dead blood vessels are replaced by the body, but always closer to the surface, so Carol's red souvenir is the visible criss-crossing of new blood vessels.

"This mark could be removed by plastic surgery, but I don't want any more operations," Carol says forcefully.

After her week of post-surgery hospitalization, Carol returned to West Texas where her husband was pressed into service, changing her bandages and applying soothing salve. Carol's instructions from the surgeon were to do anything that didn't hurt too much. In his view, the best exercise was the back-and-forth maneuvering of a vacuum cleaner. Combing and brushing hair was another suggested therapy.

"About the most vigorous thing I did was walk my three cocker spaniels," she recalls. "How they did jerk against the leashes!"

Winter was her time for recuperation, and by spring Carol was swimming laps and teaching a Red Cross life saving class.

The Dallas surgeon had warned Carol not to get pregnant, but at the same time he spoke of other of his mastectomy patients who had survived pregnancies. Carol suspected his advice was the standard safety precaution, and that he did not truly fear her cancer would return.

Carol and her husband began adoption proceedings. What a jolt to discover that in Texas, a cancer patient had to be "clean" (their word) for five years before a child could be placed in the family!

Carol panicked, fretting, "By then I'd be thirty, and they'd probably tell me I was too old to be an adoptive mother.

"Well, I got mad, and about two years after my mastectomy I quit taking precautions. I had a beautiful baby girl. When she was a year old, I realized I didn't want her to be an only child—I'd grown up as an only child and was lonely. So I had a baby boy.

"After both births I had a sixth-week checkup with the

Dallas surgeon. The second time he scolded, 'I do believe we'd better not do this again.'

"I assured him that, since I already had one child of each kind, I didn't intend to do it again."

Carol continued to consult the Dallas surgeon annually, and three times she weathered scares. Twice cysts on her back, where elastic chafed, were removed and judged benign. A lump on the right lobe of her thyroid necessitated a thyroidectomy. Fortunately, the left lobe continues to produce sufficient thyroxin so that "thyroid pills" never have been prescribed, although the earlier radium treatment had been aimed very close to the thyroid.

To refer to these three experiences as "scares" is not fair to Carol, whose policy is to wait and see, to have an ornery growth removed, to go on about her business. . . .

"Had any of those lumps been malignant, I would have taken it from there. No need to borrow trouble. It is my husband who looks on the dark side and expects the worst." Her grin is wide.

She is cheerful always; she sees no cause for gloom. She is a survivor.

1955

JANET

The year was 1955. Despite a wide friendship among women at work, in church, and in the Order of the Eastern Star, a Masonic affiliate, Janet could name not one who had undergone breast surgery. If the operation was emerging from closet secrecy, it was not yet a topic of general conversation.

Janet, a frisky wisp of a woman, was forty-eight when, toweling after a bath, she sensed that both breasts did not feel alike. Was one more flexible than the other?

Alarmed, still standing in the tub, still wet from the waist down, Janet began to examine her breasts. The technique she used was dredged up from memory. Years earlier she had read a magazine article about breast self-examination, BSE.

Never before had she checked her breasts.

What a shock when her probing fingers located a tiny, hard lump, deep in her flesh!

That was a Saturday morning.

On Monday afternoon, Janet was consulting a doctor whom she never before had met. A creature of constant good health, she had not sought medical advice in years.

The doctor promptly located the lump.

"Say, we can't let that go," he judged. "Ninety-nine chances out of a hundred, it's not malignant, but we'll have to find out for sure. I want you to enter the hospital this evening, for a biopsy tomorrow."

Tomorrow! The world was spinning too fast.

Janet returned to her office to inform co-workers, then went shopping to buy new pajamas and a robe. Dutifully, she entered the hospital and underwent surgery.

In 1955, no pathologist practiced in our city. It was Janet's husband who delivered the specimen to a laboratory fifty miles away.

Having done so, he returned to work.

The report was issued Tuesday afternoon.

In her hospital room, her doctor told Janet, "A cancer the size of a pea was detected in the center of the growth I removed. You know what that means, don't you?"

The room swirled. Janet whispered, "Yes."

"I will not leave a stone unturned," he promised. "We have to get all of this out, if at all possible, so it will be a radical mastectomy."

Janet nodded. By profession she, too, was a scientist. She could maintain a level head now.

The doctor informed her, "I will clean out all of the fatty tissue under the skin of the right breast. The lymph nodes will go, and so will the large chest muscle.

"You will be in the hospital ten days to two weeks," he continued, "and out of work at least a month. I will give you exercises while you are in the hospital so you can regain the use of your arm. Before you leave the hospital, I want you to be able to reach around behind your neck with your right arm, and touch your left ear."

Janet mused to herself that this ear touching was a silly goal. How could a movement so simple be worthy of attention?

She entered the operating room on Wednesday morning full of confidence, with no fear. Hadn't the doctor promised to leave no stone unturned? Hadn't he promised that, with exercises, she would return to normal? She knew that she was going to be all right.

Her religious faith, too, was constant.

The morning after surgery, Janet awoke and combed her hair with her right hand. Oh, it hurt, but when she lowered her arm the pain went away. With curiosity, she reached her right arm behind her neck and touched her left ear.

Why all the fuss? she wondered.

Astonished and impressed, the doctor never did assign exercises for her.

"But I knew I had to keep using that arm," Janet remembers. "I forced myself always to reach with my right arm, never my left. I reached and reached, until pain stopped me."

Her recovery was so rapid that in nine days, the doctor decided, "I'm going to send you home."

"When can I drive?" Janet asked.

"Why drive?" he countered.

"Well, you told me I have to take X-ray treatment five days a week, and I certainly won't ask anybody to chauffeur me around."

The doctor hesitated. "Don't drive before Monday." This was a reluctant concession.

So on Monday morning, twelve days after the radical mastectomy, Janet drove her husband to work, drove home, drove downtown for treatment, drove home. . . .

Alone in the car, she savored the memory of her homecoming the previous afternoon. A good neighbor arrived, delivering dinner.

"You're ironing!" the neighbor wailed, almost dropping the casserole. "I don't think you're supposed to do that."

"I don't have time to stay in bed," Janet replied briskly.

Her enforced holiday from work was a boon to Janet. After X-ray treatments, the major part of her day remained, hours she spent visiting shut-ins, housekeeping, reading. . . . It was a time for catching up.

In 1955 in our small city, the follow-up treatment for mastectomy remained chest X ray, to catch and kill any stray cancer cells. Janet received twenty-five chest X rays and ten abdominal X rays, the latter to put an end to her menstruation.

Janet continued in the vanguard of mastectomy patients, returning to work in less than a month. She was somewhat apprehensive; at least one male co-worker had always thrived on voicing sexy innuendoes.

"If anybody makes comments I don't like, I'll be ready for him," she promised herself. She was prepared to say, "You look and you look until you're through, and then have it over with."

Her peppery defense went unspoken: At the office, nobody leered. Nobody expressed curiosity. Nobody ever spoke of cancer or mastectomy.

What Janet's co-workers said was, "How are you?" and "We missed you."

She was relieved and grateful.

Away from the office, mastectomy never was a hush-hush topic with Janet. She makes no secret of her surgery, if what she reveals can help other women. She was one of our city's first volunteer visitors for Reach to Recovery.

"Reach to Recovery has been a most pleasant experience for me," Janet says. "What a reward to have a patient say to me that I did her a world of good, that merely seeing me 'not acting handicapped' boosted her morale and was an inspiration."

Lucky as she was, Janet did not escape mastectomy without post-surgery symptoms. Twenty-five years later, deep breathing continues to hurt her chest. The hard line of her incision pulls when her ribs expand.

Janet's arm did not swell for five years after surgery, and when it did, her doctor was surprised. When swelling occurs, it usually starts sooner.

"We'll send you to physical therapy to pump all that juice out," the doctor declared cheerily. Six days a week, for two weeks, Janet inserted her enlarged arm into the sleeve of a machine designed for that purpose. When the swelling receded, she was measured for her first "Jobst sleeve," a tight elastic casing from her hand to her shoulder. The sleeve was to be washed every night and replaced once a year.

Because her arm swells without it, Janet wears her Jobst sleeve every waking hour. Overnight, she wears an older sleeve, its elasticity somewhat tired, and an Ace bandage wrapped tightly around her hand. In bed, she props her arm on a pillow.

"None of this is uncomfortable, and I don't think much about it," Janet reflects. Unconcerned, she adds, "I'll probably be wearing a sleeve the rest of my life."

Janet's normal calm was ruffled, however, over the problems of prostheses. Her first breast form, an expensive, purchased one, was silicone filled. In time the silicone congealed, leaving Janet with "pebbles" inside a flesh-colored casing.

Janet slit the casing open, knocked out the pebbles, and stuffed the casing with bits of sponge and cotton and "I don't remember what all" until it seemed well-shaped and firm. It is this homemade prosthesis that she wears by choice.

Now in her seventies, Janet remains peppy, peppery, and physically active. She does her own housework. She pushes a manual lawn mower. She trims hedges. She plants and weeds flower beds.

In performing the yard chores which she loves, she guards against punctures and other injuries to her right arm and hand. Infection here does not heal itself; the infection-fighting lymph nodes were cut out in surgery. Infection in the arm is, of necessity, treated with antibiotics.

Janet never allowed mastectomy to slow her down, or to alter her life in any way. At the time of surgery she was "going through the chairs" at Eastern Star, and she continued her route to Worthy Matron with all its responsibilities and demands on her time.

"Sometimes I slept only five hours a night," she remembers.

She is riled only by people who pamper her, worrying, "Oh, don't lift that! You'll hurt your arm."

"I can do anything anybody else can," she insists spunkily.

1962

LORETTA

In 1962, at the age of forty-nine, Loretta suffered chest discomfort and suspected her heart. The Friday morning on which she was to consult her local doctor, she poked at her left breast, trying to pinpoint the exact location of the mysterious pain.

Her probing fingers discovered a lump.

She kept mute about the lump until her heart tests were complete.

"It can't be your heart," the doctor argued, perplexed. "I don't know what it is."

"How about this?" Nervously Loretta indicated the worrisome spot.

The doctor examined it and said, "Now, this is serious." He continued his exploration, probing both breasts, both underarms, both upper arms.

"I can't see that it has spread," he announced. "Now I want you to see a surgeon."

Loretta went home to debate the situation with her husband, and together they decided that the place for her was the Mayo Clinic in Rochester, Minnesota. In Loretta's large family, treatment at Mayo's was a tradition, despite the extensive travel distances involved. Loretta arranged for her admission by telephone, then spent a reflective weekend with her husband counting her blessings and bolstering her faith.

On Monday, just three days after her discovery of the lump, she and her sister flew to Rochester. On Tuesday, the Mayo Clinic doctor discovered a second lump, a much smaller one in Loretta's other breast.

Two cancers? Oh, it couldn't be!

Testing continued all week.

On the next Monday, both lumps were biopsied. The

lump on the left definitely was cancer, and that breast was removed. Tests on the right lump were inconclusive, necessitating further study.

Loretta awoke from anesthesia to hear, "Don't move that arm!" Her left arm was stretched straight out from her shoulder, and supported on a pillow.

"I had full use of my arm from the very beginning," Loretta recalls. "This I credit to the way my arm was positioned after surgery."

She learned that the cancer of her left breast had spread to her lymph nodes, and that she would remain in Rochester for treatment. In 1962 the favored treatment remained X ray; cobalt radiation was reserved mainly for deeper cancers, like that of the stomach.

Continuing laboratory tests picked up a malignancy in the material extracted from Loretta's right breast. Ten days after her first surgery, Loretta underwent a second radical mastectomy.

She recovered quickly.

When another ten days had elapsed, the X-ray procedures began. Loretta rebelled at the suggested six-week program. By necessity she now was alone in Rochester. She missed her husband. And she was homesick.

Finally it was arranged that if she remained in the hospital, and if she could tolerate double dosages of X ray, she could complete the program in three weeks.

She managed without any signs of illness.

After the three days of observation that followed her last treatment, she was allowed to fly home.

Home never looked so good!

As she undressed for bed that night, Loretta told her husband, "I'm not very pretty."

"That doesn't matter," he said emphatically. "I've got you. That's what matters."

Never again did the couple discuss Loretta's flatness.

Nor did they speak again of cancer. They went on with their lives.

"My mastectomies didn't change our lives in any way," Loretta insists.

A sister agrees, recalling that "She did beautifully, accepting the doctors' judgments in every respect."

Loretta heeded Mayo's admonition against sleeping on her sides, with its inherent risk of putting weight and pressure on her arms. Nor could she sleep on her stomach; her chest was too raw. The only possible sleeping position was flat on her back, her arms propped on pillows.

On the Friday of her homecoming week, Loretta went to visit co-workers, figuring to get the chatter behind her so that when she returned to the office on Monday, she and everybody else could concentrate on work. So congenial was the reunion that Loretta stayed downtown for three hours.

The price she paid for her socializing was a shockingly swollen right arm.

"I was terrified," she recalls. "Nobody had warned me that swelling might occur if I didn't keep my arms propped high." Via an S.O.S. telephone call to the Mayo Clinic, Loretta learned how to treat herself: by wrapping an Ace bandage tightly from her wrist to her shoulder.

She reported to work on schedule, her arm wrapped. Whenever possible she elevated the arm, giving trapped fluids the opportunity to flow from her arm back into her body where retained sections of the lymphatic system dealt with them in the body's normal fashion.

Loretta was not quite content with her progress. After four months at home, she returned to Mayo's.

There, the first goal was to return her arm to its normal size. For this, she inserted her swollen arm into the sleeve of a Jobst machine. The sleeve was inflated and deflated alternately, pumping away trapped fluids.

When her affected arm reached its normal size, both arms

were measured for tight-fitting elastic sleeves, designed to minimize swelling. She was supplied as well with instructions for massage and exercises to be done at home, and she was provided with two wooden contraptions to use in bed, one to support each arm. They folded for storage.

"My arms wouldn't stay put on those boards," she recalls with laughter. "They just kept sliding off. But I kept working at it, and I used those boards for years."

The years did pass. Loretta's right arm quit swelling and aching. Eureka? No such luck. The annoying symptoms merely switched to her left arm.

She confides, "I find that if I don't keep using my arms—if I don't work them hard—the swelling and aching increases. I keep very active physically. Aquacize helps a great deal."

When Loretta lost her breasts to cancer, a beloved niece was fifteen, with brand-new breasts. The nature of Loretta's surgery troubled the girl greatly.

Although cancer has been common in Loretta's large family, hers is the only known case of breast cancer. Her sisters, however, all suffer fibrocystic disease and are ever watchful for out-of-the-ordinary lumps and thickenings.

Loretta's first prostheses were purchased at a medical supply shop and were, in her words, "so miserably heavy that the straps of my bra dug painfully into my shoulders." Loretta next tried a blow-up brassiere, light as a cloud, but with the unfortunate tendency to float high when she raised her arms; there was nothing to secure the bra in place.

Next she padded her pre-surgery bras, adding the weight of fishermen's lead sinkers for anchors.

After thirteen years of "making do," and never being satisfied, Loretta was fitted in a department store with prostheses that are weighted but not burdensomely heavy. Inserted in a brassiere of the same brand as the prostheses, they delight Loretta. "They are comfortable, they stay in place, they look natural—and I love them!" she reports.

Shopping can be difficult for a mastectomee. Loretta

recalls her first excursion after surgery. "I tried to push hangers across a rod, and I couldn't! It was then that I was totally aware that my pectoral muscles—my push-and-pull muscles—were gone."

Fifteen years after surgery, she still couldn't wear dresses with slim sleeves because one arm or the other remained swollen. Gradually the swelling abated, until now she is virtually unlimited in her choice of clothes, and her arms stay soft and pain-free.

To discourage swelling, Loretta still wears the elastic sleeves around the house. She is now retired from her secretarial job.

She is alert to sudden fever and a sore arm, signs of infection. Three times these symptoms have occurred without any outward sign of injury—no infected hangnail, no cut, no bruise. In every case the infection was rapidly cured by antibiotics.

Loretta discounts annoyances.

"I'd have radical surgery again, if I had to make the choice again," she insists. "Life is the most important thing, not breasts."

1965

FRANNY

"Four and a half hours of savage butchery, killing a gnat with a sledgehammer," is how Franny describes her radical mastectomy in 1965. She was forty-four years old.

Her cancer was the size of a match head. To treat it, all breast tissue was removed, plus the lymph nodes, plus muscle to the bone. Scars remain visible on X rays where her bone was scraped during mastectomy.

But the breast surgery itself was just the introduction to her troubles, and in comparison, a minor irritant. A skin graft and a blood transfusion caused the greatest difficulties.

Franny's own breast skin was judged too thin to seal her newly flat chest, so the surgeon fashioned a patch with skin removed from her thigh, leaving her thigh tender and slow to heal. The graft did not completely "take," and the rotting flesh on her chest emitted putrid odors close to unbearable. Healing continued slowly even after "pinch grafts" replaced the dead matter.

Even worse than Franny's colossal case of body odor was her serum hepatitis, caused by the blood transfusion. This put her back in the hospital for a month.

It wasn't until five months after the mastectomy that she was judged sufficiently recovered to undergo the then-common operation for menstruating women who had breast cancer—an oophorectomy. Oophorectomy is the surgical removal of the ovaries, to halt the ovaries' production of hormones.

(Today oophorectomies usually are not performed on menstruating women without cancer involvement in their lymph nodes. Also, blood testing methods are now so sophisticated that hepatitis from transfusion is rare indeed.)

Her instant menopause caused Franny to suffer extreme

hot flashes and sweats which continued for thirteen years, until her doctor prescribed an estrogen cream.

"I wasn't going to let feeling punk make an invalid out of me," she recalls. In stubborn determination she raised her own children and a child not her own. She illustrated seven books for major publishers with a mastectomy-affected arm that swells and hurts. Magazine stories and books carry her by-line.

Franny's mastectomy story began in her physician's office, during a regular physical examination. The doctor asked, "Do you have a scar on this breast?"

"Not that I know of," she replied, puzzled.

"I don't remember it. Let's have it X-rayed."

"Is it a lump?" Franny's voice trembled. She knew the significance of breast lumps.

"More like a dimple," the doctor replied.

The tiny, hard to see depression was three-fourths of an inch from the nipple of Franny's left breast, at ten o'clock.

X-rays, the technique of cancer screening at the time, read out negative.

"But I still want this biopsied," the doctor insisted.

Franny fumed at the cost in money and time. It was December; she had too much to do. There just wasn't space on her agenda for a hospital procedure, however short.

Her Girl Scout troop was to make plywood hot-pot mats for Christmas gifts. Franny prepared the materials and set up card tables and chairs in her home for the next meeting. That would be one less chore to perform when she returned from the hospital after the biopsy, after receiving the good news which she fully expected. The possibility that her "dimple" might be the tug of cancer did not enter her thinking. She was just too busy to have cancer!

If the mothers of Girl Scouts received hot-pot mats that Christmas, it was not by Franny's guidance.

The biopsy on Friday seemed to go well. When Franny

awoke from anesthesia, her husband was at her bedside, grinning.

Franny looked down and saw only a square patch of a bandage on her breast. Had cancer gained a foothold, the breast would have been gone.

"See, I told you," Franny challenged in glee.

On Saturday morning, her doctor signed her release but requested that she stay in the hospital until afternoon "to be sure the anesthetic has worn off." Her husband, there to drive her home, returned home alone to tend their two young children.

He returned to her room unexpectedly, at 11:30 A.M.

"You're too early," Franny scolded.

Her doctor appeared on her husband's heels, admitting, "I sent for him." He sat on her bed and reached for her hand.

Oh, no! *Oh, no! Oh, no!* Every cell in her body cried out against the news she knew was coming.

The pathologist, performing one last test, had found a cancer the size of a match head. A radical mastectomy was the standard treatment of the time.

Stunned, Franny rejected the news. Cancer? It couldn't be true! So extreme was her reaction that tranquilizers were administered to her regularly until the Monday surgery.

Her parents-in-law were summoned to care for the children.

Following the four and one-half hour surgery, Franny remembers awakening off and on with a desire to go to the bathroom, and being told to lie still. Nurses in white uniforms paraded through her room. Her strength came from her husband, ever attentive beside her bed.

On the third day after surgery, the full impact of what had happened hit Franny. Rebellious, bitter thoughts pounded at her. Wasn't nursing an infant supposed to make a woman almost immune to breast cancer? She had nursed one baby for eight months, the other for nine months.

With anger motivating her, she demanded of the doctor, "What are my chances of getting cancer someplace else?"

"No greater than before," he assured her, "except for the other breast which we will watch carefully." He suggested that after five years, the increased risk would end.

Spending Christmas at home, her first hospital interlude over, Franny no longer rebelled against the operation's cost in money and time. She was content to be with her family, rejoicing that the cancer had been found early. She would be around to light the tree next Christmas and the next. And she would live to see grandchildren at the tree.

As indeed she did, because of the dimple that was the early clue to cancer.

Franny's lymph nodes had shown suspicious changes but no cancer, and after some debate the doctors decided to "leave no stone unturned" in curing her.

In cases of earlier date, described previously, X ray was used. One patient also was treated with radium. By 1965 cobalt radiation apparently was the treatment of choice for breast cancer. Cobalt was ordered for Franny.

When, after the fifteenth treatment, she began to vomit, she assumed that the radiation was to blame.

Then she turned yellow.

Hepatitis!

Its treatment put Franny back in the hospital for an entire month. During this interlude Franny took stock. She did have a choice. Either she could live her life in tormented fear of cancer or she could move forward normally, confident that cancer would never return.

She chose the second path.

She resumed illustrating, free lance.

"The day I received my first check from work I'd done while ill was a real milestone," she remembers.

Yes, Franny was confident, but she wasn't foolhardy. A suspected dimple in her remaining breast sent her rushing in panic to the doctor. No problem. Then two years after her mastectomy the doctor discovered a lump, a suspected milk gland. Yet it merited biopsy.

The operating theaters were booked for a solid week. Franny had to wait her turn.

Oh, the turmoil of that week! Oh, the agony! Franny began by telling herself that the lump was benign, but by midweek she was in anguish, certain that she was again dealing with cancer.

This time when she awakened from anesthesia, the bandage on her chest was bulky.

"So it's gone," she said resignedly.

"No, it isn't," her husband replied. "It was a milk gland, exactly as expected."

Beginning then, Franny became ambivalent about her six-month checkups, afraid of what the doctor might find, afraid not to let him search.

But fear is only occasionally her companion. She says, "I could be hit by a car while crossing a street, but I won't quit crossing streets. I could get cancer again, perhaps, but I won't quit planning the future. I'm a living proof that cancer caught in time can be cured."

1971

CHRISTY

Pre-surgery dialogue is etched so sharply in Christy's mind that, ten years later, she can repeat it verbatim.

She tells it in her own words:

During my regular yearly checkup with my gynecologist, I was lying relaxed on the table rather enjoying the sensuous feel of his hands moving over my breasts. Suddenly I realized he had stopped at one place. He poked at it again, then turned to a nearby table.

I raised on an elbow to see what he was doing.

On my chart sheet, he drew a quick sketch. Two smiles. Two dots. Then an X.

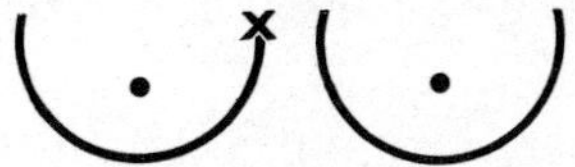

"X marks the spot," I said, stretching for a joke.

"I don't think it's anything," he said. "But in this location, upper inner quadrant, well, it's the most dangerous spot for a malignancy. Can't fool around with that."

Ten minutes later I was down the hall in the same medical building, in my surgeon's office. He was jabbing at the spot.

"I really think we ought to biopsy this right away," he said. "However, I'm leaving on vacation tomorrow and won't be back for several weeks."

"What do you think I should do?" Fear made my voice shake.

He frowned. "You never can tell when water will run over the dam."

I knew exactly what he meant: You never can tell when a cell will break loose from the primary cancer and seed elsewhere in the body.

Inside me everything congealed into a hot, tight knot. It hurt to breathe.

"This shouldn't wait," he emphasized. "You had better find another surgeon."

Nearly in tears from suddenly facing this unknown horror, I fled back to the hospital laboratory where I work. I needed advice from a doctor I could trust, and who better than the pathologist I worked with daily?

He pondered my problem, then suggested, "If you're willing, I'll make the arrangements."

Relief flooded through me. All I wanted was to hand the whole problem over to someone else, like a child handing problems to parents, expecting everything to turn out all right.

I slipped into my lab coat and went back to my hospital chores, trying to shove all the if's, maybe's, and but's out of my mind.

A few hours later, a young, brash, bearded doctor breezed into the lab.

"It looks like it's going to be you and me, Babe," he announced.

You and me? I stared at him, bewildered and unbelieving. He was our new hot-shot surgeon, a specialist, on the staff only a few months. He was hot-tempered (maybe so was I) and already the two of us had locked horns.

"We've got a date Friday morning," he told me, cheerily.

What had my friend, the pathologist, gotten me into? Oh, I knew the man had a fine reputation as a surgeon, but what about our personality clash? I yearned for my familiar, middle-aged, clean-shaven, comfortable surgeon. Oh, what an ill-timed vacation he was taking!

"Do you want to poke at the lump now?" I offered obediently.

"Plenty of time for that," he said. "Go get a mammogram and have them send me the report, and I'll see you later."

The mammogram was negative. Oh, joy! And I couldn't locate the offending lump, even though I knew exactly where it was supposed to be. My breasts were large and fleshy; but still, you'd think I could find the spot two doctors had prodded!

Maybe it had dissolved, all by itself.

Thursday afternoon I left the lab and walked around the corner to the surgery wing where I signed a surgery permit. It read, "Breast Biopsy, Radical Mastectomy if Malignant."

I felt the world was spinning in altogether the wrong direction.

I slept that night in the hospital where I worked, suddenly no longer behind-the-scenes. Now I was a patient.

The reality took getting used to.

So did the reality of Friday morning in the operating theater.

I awoke from the anesthetic feeling tied down by a dozen straps and tubes. Over my head hung a bag of blood. "A neg" I read to myself. "They got the right type."

No one had to inform me how the biopsy came out: The blood bag told me.

Right then I became an ostrich. It was done—my breast was gone. It was an accomplished fact. The small "inner upper quadrant" lump (in a dangerous place) had been malignant. Who knew "if the water had gone over the dam?" Who knew the future?

Measured in months and years, how much "future" did I have?

How I wished the doctors had guarded their tongues! Did they know how much additional anguish they cause by cheerful but careless comments like that "over the dam" parallel?

My husband brought my small soft comforter from home and tucked it around me. He knew I always felt a little cold in the hospital.

I felt his love in the comforter's warmth.

The hospital days of recovery are substantially blocked from my memory. I was in a familiar place, surrounded by friends and co-workers who took care of me and eased my pain.

Six weeks later I was back in the lab, again on the hospital staff, no longer a patient.

By now, I've almost forgotten the long silvery-looking incision reaching from my armpit almost to my navel, the months of wearing sterile surgical gauze over the few places that were slow in healing, the numbness of my skin on my back and chest where nerves were cut and skin was stretched taut.

I've about forgotten lying on the table while the cobalt machine ticked away the seconds above me. Was this worth the chance of future radiation-related sickness? Or was my chance better to let the cobalt radiation hunt down any remaining malignant cells? Would I have been better off with chemotherapy? Or with no therapy at all?

Two years passed.

Then I developed endometriosis, the cells which normally lined the uterus spilling into my abdominal cavity. This, combined with an enlarged uterus, made a hysterectomy imperative.

Of course, because of my cancer history, I could not take hormones to ease the hysterectomy-caused instant menopause. Consequently, I suffered sweats and hot flashes.

Mammograms were old hat to me. Long before my mastectomy, my doctor had requested regular X rays of the breast because my breast tissue was so extensive. He believed a manual exam was inadequate to find lumps.

So there I was again with the radiologist, four years after my mastectomy and two years after the hysterectomy. He was examining me, and I had a horrible feeling of history repeating itself. I braced for the worst even before the radiologist got to a certain spot and stopped.

"You found something," I accused.

"This is the same little spot as last year," he reported calmly. "We've been watching it."

The same little spot as last year! I seethed with anger. This is my life! I deserve to know what's happening in my body!

There were three routes open to me, the radiologist said.

First, a biopsy, taking no further action if the biopsy tested negative.

Second, a simple mastectomy even though the biopsy tested negative.

Third, a radical mastectomy if the biopsy tested positive.

Over this third possibility, I didn't cringe. If there was cancer, I wanted the breast gone.

Indeed the third possibility was in God's hands, not mine.

But the first and second options—oh, how could I choose between them? Did I have the courage to give up my remaining breast if I didn't absolutely have to? Conversely, did I have the courage to continue living with a breast that sent out signals of trouble?

I phoned my husband, and we met for lunch in a pleasant restaurant. We might have fled to the privacy of our own home for this vital discussion, but oddly I craved impersonal surroundings.

We drank beer with our meal, a rare mid-day naughtiness. The meal evolved into a celebration of a sort.

We discussed our options.

To have options was a new experience for us. No choice had been involved in the two previous surgeries. They had had to be done.

Clearheaded, but with agony, we arrived at a decision. I would have a simple mastectomy even if the lump tested negative. With the second breast gone, our continuing worry about breast cancer would be ended.

And this came to pass.

The lump, biopsied, was negative, while the breast tissue itself showed dangerous pre-cancerous changes. We had been wise to opt for the mastectomy.

Oddly, although the surgery was less extensive, my second mastectomy was the more traumatic. I was kept in the hospital longer. It took me longer to get back on my feet.

I am alive and grateful!

The field of breast cancer therapy is changing rapidly. This I know from hospital chat, not from my own research, for I still can't spot a breast cancer article in a medical journal without a quick pulse of panic. How fast I pass these articles by!

Neither do I read books about cancer of any sort.

My annual physical examinations create apprehension in me. *What next? What next?*

I'm fifty-five, overweight, and my front looks like a disaster area: radical mastectomy scar on the right, simple mastectomy scar on the left, total hysterectomy scar down the center.

How does this affect my life, and the lives of women like me? I have given the question a lot of introspective thought.

You never get over the awareness of your mortality. You learn to appreciate every day that dawns, rain or shine, cold or hot. You don't care much about things that once seemed so important: house, clothes, money, doodads.

And, most of all, you appreciate the family that sticks close to you, the children who keep in close contact, the husband who still tucks you in—and in spite of it all, still chases you around the bedroom once in a while.

1972

GLORIA

Her surgeon removed the bandages, and Gloria looked down at her still-angry, still-tender scar.

She scoffed, "What fifty-year-old widow is going around showing this to anybody?" That was in 1972.

Within a few years she had a suitor. She appealed to the surgeon, "What should I tell him?"

"Tell him you had cancer," the surgeon said briskly. "Tell him you are cured."

You are cured. Such beautiful words!

Gloria's first lump had appeared suddenly on her left breast. It was a cyst which the surgeon drained in his office.

"This is not cancer," he told her immediately. "Tumors aren't filled with fluid. However, I think this should come out. It'll just fill up again if we don't get rid of it."

"O.K.," Gloria agreed. She was about to dress when the surgeon called, "Wait a minute. I haven't checked your other side."

Examining her right breast, he said in concern, "There is something here."

She entered the hospital. Her biopsy tested positive. Her right breast was removed.

The pain was not overwhelming, and no narcotics were administered. What troubled Gloria more than chest discomfort was her arm. During surgery it had been wrapped tightly, from shoulder to palm of hand, with a sticky adhesive tape that looked something like an Ace bandage. The purpose of the wrapping was to eliminate swelling.

For six months, Gloria experienced a love-hate relationship with the binding. She felt better because of it, but its tightness and hotness caused agony. It pinched when she bent her elbow. The necessity to keep it dry made bathing awkward. As it soiled, it offended Gloria's sensibilities.

During her recovery days in the hospital, Gloria was calm and happy. Her cancer had been caught early, before it invaded the lymph nodes. She would need neither radiation nor chemotherapy. Her future looked bright.

Ten days after the mastectomy of her right breast, Gloria was told the left breast needed to come off, too, because of fibrocystic disease. Otherwise she would face hospitalization after hospitalization, biopsy after biopsy. Growths were sure to recur.

Between her first mastectomy in March and her second in July, Gloria didn't brood. By the end of April she was bowling in a tournament 200 miles from home, with her surgeon's approval. The absence of her right breast didn't affect her right-handed bowling.

Gloria's left breast, removed in July, showed no cancer. The benign growths in it were described as "clusters of grapes."

While she was under anesthetic for this second surgery, Gloria's right arm was rewrapped. Her left arm remained unwrapped and unswollen, the left mastectomy having been "simple," the right mastectomy "radical," with removal of lymph glands and chest muscle.

Gloria wore the tight wrapping for six months, and when it finally was removed, her flesh was marked with raw, red rings.

Free of the binding, Gloria plunged into exercise to regain full strength in her arm. Swelling came and went, sometimes noted in the mirror, sometimes obvious when she struggled to button cuffs.

Gloria walked then, and she continues to walk now for exercise, despite the certainty that her arm will swell. Fluids in the arm cannot be removed normally via the lymphatic drainage system; the lymph is gone. So the fluids remain, puffing the arm and causing mild discomfort.

"The surgeon wants me to bend my elbow and carry my arm waist-high," Gloria confides, "but I just can't step out briskly without swinging my arms!" So she endures the swelling that comes after a long walk.

In common with other mastectomees, she habitually props her arm high to aid drainage by gravity.

Another function of the lymph is to remove bacteria and certain proteins from the tissues. Exactly one year after her first mastectomy, Gloria was dressing for work when she noticed a bright red spot on the back of her arm. How peculiar. . . . There was no cut or scrape to explain the symptom.

Within an hour of her arrival at work, her entire arm was fire-red, with a frightening white streak running its length.

Shivering, her teeth chattering, feeling totally miserable, she drove herself to the surgeon's office.

"I'm going to put you in the hospital," he told her.

"No!" She refused hospitalization.

An antibiotic cured the infection.

On two more occasions, years apart, Gloria's arm erupted in a measles-type rash. Now she carries antibiotics wherever she goes, for emergency use.

"I've got one complaint and only one," Gloria reveals. "I'm really disturbed that my surgeon didn't warn me about what might happen. He never said swelling might plague me forever. He never suggested that infection might strike. He never hinted that nerves severed in surgery would continue to nag me.

"I can handle whatever comes, but I prefer to know ahead of time what to expect."

No complaints shadowed Gloria's post-surgery hospital days, which she remembers as emotionally untroubled. Months passed before depression set in. Then she fretted, *Might cancer strike again?*

Years later she was asking herself, "Why did it have to be done? Why isn't there a substitute for amputation?"

She is aware that the passing years have brought changes in mastectomy technique. When possible, surgeons carve less deeply. Most of today's mastectomees are less disfigured and less handicapped than those of the past.

Too, a new stress on physical therapy hastens the woman's full use of her arm. (No exercises were assigned to Gloria; she worked out a program by herself, guessing it crucial to her well-being.)

Nowadays, Reach to Recovery volunteers, at the surgeon's request, appear at hospital bedsides as living proof that women return to normal after mastectomy. No longer is mastectomy a secret.

Gloria herself is a Reach to Recovery volunteer, a hospital auxiliary volunteer, and a member of One Day at a Time. The path of her life has not been altered by mastectomy; she still plans to work until retirement age. She travels. She dates. She sews. She tends her lawn and home. She bowls twice weekly.

It is only occasionally that she mourns her missing breasts. Her prostheses are comfortable; she is confident that she looks "normal." She ascribes her occasional blues to the reality of cancer hitting home.

1976

YVONNE

Yvonne always had been aware that her small breasts were lumpy. About this, no doctor had expressed concern, nor put a name to the condition.

It was her husband who noticed the new flaw, a pea-shaped lump different from the others. Yvonne was thirty-seven.

She sought prompt medical counsel, motivated by the premature heart-attack death of a friend. Her internist ordered mammograms, her first ever.

Within a week, and before her mammogram appointment, the pea-shaped lump disappeared. Apparently it had been a cyst that drained itself.

Yvonne's mammograms showed calcification within the ducts, unusually severe in a woman not yet forty. While the condition itself was not cancerous, it could hide a cancer.

Yvonne was to enter into a period of very careful watching, by herself, by her internist, and by the radiologist. Her next mammogram was scheduled in three months.

But her husband was not comfortable with the "wait and watch" prescription. He favored biopsy to end the uncertainty. Together he and Yvonne went to consult the internist.

Of concern was the fact that, after Yvonne quit nursing her third baby, her breasts remained hard and lumpy, knottier than ever before. And they were sore all the time.

The internist judged that a biopsy was not justified. If all of Yvonne's lumps were removed, there would be scant breast tissue left! To examine only six or eight lumps would risk missing one vital clue.

Yvonne recalls the internist's saying, in extreme casualness, "You could have bilateral simple mastectomies." Having voiced this idea, he went on to discuss other matters.

Yvonne translated his comment to mean, "If you can't handle the uncertainty of these lumps, you can have your breasts removed."

Still young, and joyfully married, she didn't want her breasts removed! Nor did she want to appear less than a totally cooperative patient.

As instructed, she waited and watched for three months. Her March mammogram showed no change.

It was during April that changes became obvious. Her left breast, always the larger, was drawing in and shrinking. Now it was smaller than the right breast. A flat, disk-shaped growth on the left breast had become harder, and as big as a quarter.

The medical advice again was to wait and watch.

Yvonne's June mammogram again showed no change, but this time the radiologist on duty was a different man, and he expressed uneasiness. As his fingers probed her breasts, he said, "I don't like what I see, and I don't like what I feel."

By this time, the hard disk on her left breast was as large as a half dollar, and radiating flashes of pain. All the doctors agreed that this was not cancer, and a later biopsy proved them right.

The cancer was elsewhere.

"If you were my wife or daughter," the radiologist said, "I would insist on a biopsy."

A biopsy was what Yvonne's husband had been pushing for from the beginning.

"No need to rush," the radiologist consoled. "Take your time."

Now, for the first time, Yvonne consulted a surgeon.

The surgeon suggested three alternatives, in reverse order of his recommendation.

First, biopsies of both breasts.

Second, bilateral simple mastectomies—the removal of skin, tissue, and nipple of both breasts, leaving untouched the muscle and lymph nodes.

Third, bilateral subcutaneous mastectomy plus reconstruction, both in the same procedure. In this method a woman's own skin and nipple are retained. The muscle is bisected and the prosthesis—a silicone-filled form—is slipped between muscle layers which support it.

Voila! The woman looks the same as before. Nipples even remain sensitive to touch, if all goes well.

Yvonne opted for this procedure, although it meant hospitalization far from home. No plastic surgeon practices in our city of 30,000.

Unworried, because no doctor had urged haste, Yvonne entertained summer houseguests and scheduled her mastectomy/reconstruction for August.

August arrived. Dutifully, Yvonne traveled to a large southwestern city and reported to her plastic surgeon.

From him, she learned certain facts. The breast tissue that he removed would be examined by a pathologist while Yvonne remained on the operating table under sedation. Should any sign of cancer emerge, the plastic surgeon would "close"—stitch up her wound. Later another surgeon would take over and perform the needed radical mastectomy.

The plastic surgeon warned that with subcutaneous mastectomy there is some residual breast tissue, attached to skin and muscle. This tissue might possibly respond to hormone levels. In other words, there would be enough remaining tissue to host the most persistent of cancer cells.

Yvonne considered this danger as a distant off-chance. Hadn't all the doctors judged her breast irregularities to be benign?

With faith that all would be well, she underwent the surgery.

"All is well!" her husband told her, when she awakened. "There is no cancer. The implants are in place."

Hurrah!

The pathology report showed that Yvonne's left breast was "dangerously pre-malignant."

Yvonne dozed all day, between bouts of nausea without vomiting. She suffered constant, severe pain in her shoulders, from the way in which she had been taped for surgery. Whenever she moved, she hurt in the front from her chin to her pelvis, and her arms ached from shoulder to elbow.

"This is not painful surgery," the plastic surgeon had promised. "I will not order pain killers for you."

But with his permission, a much-needed pain pill was administered at 10 P.M.

Yvonne sat up for dinner, then was unable to cope with the standard diet her doctor had ordered. Her taste buds revolted against sugar and salt.

She prepared herself for the night, walking to the bathroom with her husband watchfully beside her. She was able to lift her arms high enough to wash her face and comb her hair, simple actions that brought on total exhaustion.

The next morning she climbed gingerly from bed and groomed herself. Weakness washed over her in waves. Bed was still the place for her, she realized.

It was one o'clock when the plastic surgeon entered Yvonne's room, announcing, "I don't know what to do with you."

"Oh?" Yvonne was wary.

The dismay of the plastic surgeon was evident. In the operating arena some twenty-four hours earlier, he had received the green light to continue. Yvonne's reconstruction was complete.

He told his patient, "The pathologist has reported the discovery of cancer in an unsuspected area of your left breast, a cancer so small that if the knife blade had sliced a hair differently in one direction, the next slice would have passed beyond it."

The surgeon was faced with a dilemma. Should the prostheses be left in place? Or should one or both be sacrificed to radical mastectomy?

"I will take this problem to the tumor board, tonight," the plastic surgeon told Yvonne.

That group of knowledgeable, experienced doctors concluded that since Yvonne's cancer was so minute, the surgery already performed should be its cure. Just in case any of the cells had strayed off, a course of chemotherapy was ordered.

Yvonne returned home to swallow dutifully her prescribed pills on five selected days of every six weeks. Each dose left her nauseated for two or three days in a type of discomfort which she describes as "one stage short of vomiting."

Yvonne rode with the punches. Rather than feeling angry or upset, she felt content, almost smug, as if she were "having her cake and eating it, too." Wasn't her cancer gone? Wasn't her figure exactly as before: Her guardian angel had guided the pathologist's hand, she was certain.

Less than four months after her mastectomies/reconstructions, and while still on chemotherapy, Yvonne noticed a spot above the bulk of her left breast, near the shoulder. It was in the upper outer quadrant, the quadrant where cancer is most common. It worried Yvonne that light reflected differently from that spot. Also, when she picked up the skin in that area and rubbed it, she sensed grittiness like grains of sand.

What should she do? Flee to the doctor? And to which of her many doctors should she flee?

Oh, she had sought medical advice so often! Might she be pegged a neurotic? This she feared.

So she postponed a medical confrontation.

The postponement was brief. Within a few days of Yvonne's own discovery, her husband noticed three or four additional spots which he described as "spongy."

He insisted that she consult the local surgeon.

From the surgeon, Yvonne learned that the blubbery spots were "fatty necrosis," the death or destruction of body tissue or cells while still in place and surrounded by living tissue. Gangrene and bed sores are also classified as "fatty necrosis."

"This condition can result from any breast trauma," the surgeon informed her, "and your surgery certainly qualifies as 'trauma.'"

She was in solid agreement with that judgment!

But the medical judgment again to "wait and watch" again was disputed by Yvonne's husband. "I want these spots biopsied yesterday," he roared. "Not tomorrow or the day after, but yesterday!"

Wilted from functioning as an intermediary between a concerned husband and delaying doctors, Yvonne suggested that he take over the patient-doctor dialogue.

The surgeon told him, "If you are that concerned, send her back in two weeks instead of four."

More blubbery spots emerged. But the most frightening event of those two waiting weeks was the rapid growth of the flaw near Yvonne's shoulder, now the size of a lima bean.

Yvonne made the long trip to the city where her plastic surgeon practiced.

He judged that the prosthesis implanted in Yvonne's left chest had broken, and that she was suffering a reaction to leaking silicone. He volunteered to mail another prosthesis to her hometown surgeon, so that he might make a trade.

What was lurking within that lima bean? Neither Yvonne nor her local surgeon were willing to wait out the vagaries of the United States Mail. They agreed on an immediate biopsy.

Again it was cancer that lurked, this time a cancer the size of the eraser on a new lead pencil. The cancer comprised one-third of the removed tissue. The other two-thirds was "fatty necrosis."

The rediscovery of cancer meant a farewell to Yvonne's reconstructed left breast. Her implanted prosthesis along with previously retained skin, nipple, tissue, lymph nodes, and muscle would have to go, to save her life.

For the necessary radical mastectomy, Yvonne returned to the major city, where consultation with cancer specialists was available and where "estrogen binding studies" could be done following surgery. Such a study alternately is called "estrogen-receptor assay." Its purpose is to determine if a cancer is stimulated in its growth and reproduction by the presence of estrogens. If it is not, there is no need for operations to cut off estrogen production.

Now Yvonne was under the care of an oncologist, a cancer specialist, who told her, "No matter what we find, I hope to buy you fifteen years."

Fifteen years would put Yvonne's youngest child into college, barely. Fifteen years were decidedly better than any fewer.

So the radical mastectomy was performed.

The pathology report showed cancer in six lymph nodes and "multiple microscopic sized spots of cancer in the breast and fatty tissue."

As a rule of thumb, the fewer lymph nodes infiltrated, the better the chance for survival.

There was not a large enough single malignant tumor to run the important "estrogen binding studies." Nonetheless, Yvonne's doctors were certain that estrogen was the culprit in her case. By this time, a doctor who specialized in cancer research had involved himself in Yvonne's case. Doctors were fairly stumbling over her! Surely their accumulated wisdom would evolve a cure!

Their accumulated wisdom advised Yvonne to undergo a bilateral oophorectomy and a bilateral adrenalectomy, both surgeries designed to stop her body from producing estrogens.

Oophorectomy. Adrenalectomy. Such big words! Oophorectomy is the surgical removal of the ovaries. Adrenalectomy is the surgical removal of two small endocrine glands, one above each kidney. These tiny glands supply ten per cent of the body's estrogens.

"Do I have to have the adrenalectomy?" Yvonne rebelled. "What if it doesn't work?"

"It jolly well better work," the oncologist said, "or you don't stand the chance of a snowball in hell."

With such odds against her, Yvonne had no choice but to return to the operating room for her fourth surgery in seven months.

Now, five years later, Yvonne is a hospital visitor for Reach to Recovery, a charter member of the local One Step at a Time, a Bosom Buddy, and an officer for the local branch of the American Cancer Society.

Her friends watch in astonishment as she teaches Sunday school and sings in the church choir, as she assumes assorted school chores which other parents are "too busy" to do, as she jogs and walks and swims, as she sews her own clothes and the children's. . . .

Is she cramming a lifetime of good works into fifteen years?

How does she manage it all? Is she bubbling with excess energy and good health?

She is not. She pushes herself.

"I'm doing everything to get back to normal, to get my body back in shape," she confides. "I'm not one to sit and rock and wait to die."

Circumstances merit rejoicing. Yvonne's right breast never developed cancer. Her reconstruction of this right breast is comfortable and "natural." Her own right nipple, after eighteen months of pain, now responds to touch all of the time, with half its previous sensation.

It is not the cancer itself nor the mastectomies that cause Yvonne's current physical problems. Rather, her troubles emerge as a result of the oophorectomy and the adrenalectomy.

Forbidden to take estrogen in any form, and restricted to low-level hydrocortisone therapies, she suffers hot flashes and embarrassing sweats. The adrenalectomy has caused Addison's disease, the symptoms of which include being unable to field physical stress with aplomb.

"I don't handle normal problems and setbacks well," she admits. "Illness, fatigue, and accidents throw me for a loop. The summer heat is nearly impossible to bear. And my joints hurt all the time."

Yvonne is self-critical, believing she has undergone a post-surgery personality change which has made her impatient and short-tempered. If this is true, she conceals it well. Friends see Yvonne as a peerless example of courage and determination. Her faith shines through.

Yvonne regrets the effect of her illness on her children. The older two became drop-outs from after-school activities, sensing that she couldn't cope with car pools. Not only did her kindergartener develop a fear of her own impending death, but she insisted that Yvonne had two breasts.

"Count them," Yvonne would challenge.

"One, TWO," the child would answer.

Cancer discussed in the media distresses all of Yvonne's children. Each of them checks and double-checks the dates of her upcoming medical examinations. They are watchdogs, assuring that she does not skip an appointment.

Near the time of each appointment, Yvonne's husband develops a "nervous stomach" and is physically ill. Except for this quirk, he has been her tower of strength, never letting her feel sorry for herself, taking a positive attitude, whatever loomed ahead.

"Nobody's life is certain," he insists. "Nobody has guarantees."

Yvonne believes that their burden was lightened tremendously because they never had to face up to a terminal illness. No doctor ever suggested that Yvonne's cancer was beyond cure.

"As I adjusted, the children did, too," Yvonne remembers. "From drop-outs, they have become drop-ins, now that I can handle more. The two younger children think it is hilarious to play catch with my prothesis—but I allow no football. I can't risk a puncture. Prostheses are too expensive!"

1976

NANCY

"That I wouldn't live to see my children grown was my biggest fear and fright," Nancy reveals. After a thoughtful pause, she giggles and adds, "And I was thinking of myself, too. I didn't want to die.

"But truly, you cling to life for the family."

In 1976, Nancy was thirty-nine years old. Her six children ranged in age from five to fifteen.

It was in October of that year when Nancy first examined her breasts, using as a guide an illustrated magazine article. Laboriously, uncertainly, she followed the sketches step by step.

"I'd always been too embarrassed to ask my doctor how to do it," she remembers ruefully. "But all of a sudden there was a spate of articles insisting BSE was the thing to do—so I thought I'd better get with it.

"Talk of beginner's luck, or whatever. . . : I noticed a funny difference in the right breast, a kind of thickening. I assured myself that a thickening wasn't a lump, and a lump was what I was hunting."

The existence of the strange thickening played on Nancy's mind but she didn't take action until ten days later when, between sets of tennis, conversation focused on a friend who was recovering from a breast biopsy. Two women present revealed that they, too, had undergone biopsies for peculiar irregularities in their breasts.

Three young women in a group of twelve! In panic, Nancy thought, *God, I'd better not mess around with this.* She completed the morning of tennis, then rushed home to telephone a surgeon. Her appointment for two o'clock that afternoon gave her time only for a fast lunch and a quick shower.

The surgeon told her, "Normally a thickening is just milk

glands. Nancy, I really think this is nothing. But let's schedule a biopsy, just to be sure."

The surgeon was correct; the thickening was not malignant. But beneath the thickening, well hidden, a cancer lurked.

Later, Nancy's surgeon reported that her lymph nodes "looked horrible to the naked eye." He was fearful that the cancer had spread far.

He performed the radical mastectomy.

Upon awakening, Nancy knew immediately that her breast was gone. Nonetheless, she asked the question of her husband.

"Yes, it is gone," he reported. Then he told her what he would repeat many, many times: that it didn't matter to him what was cut off, that it was her he loved, not her breast.

It took a lot of talking before she was convinced.

The laboratory reported that, of the lymph nodes that had appeared so threatening, only one was cancer-invaded.

It was Nancy's husband who insisted that she go to M. D. Anderson Hospital and Tumor Institute in Houston, Texas, for treatment, because a close friend, near to death, had been treated there. He lives on, his body apparently free from cancer.

Two weeks after her mastectomy, Nancy traveled to Houston with her husband. Her first chore at the hospital was to fill out a medical history in which she was asked to enumerate relatives who had had cancer.

It was then that she became poignantly aware of her hereditary risk, because her maternal grandmother had died of breast cancer. Until that moment she had forgotten what she must have read much earlier, that breast cancer tends to "run in families."

That first day at M. D. Anderson, Nancy underwent test after test, each one necessitating a wait for a complex machine. In each waiting room were other patients, and the harder Nancy tried to block out the cancer-centered conversation, the clearer she heard. And the more she overheard, the more she worried.

What drilled into her very guts was the presence of children as patients. Her own children were much on her mind.

When the day of tests ended, she returned to her motel room and phoned home.

Her five-year-old answered the telephone.

Nancy burst into tears. At that juncture, it was not in her power to reassure and comfort those at home.

Nancy expresses awe at the M. D. Anderson experience. "Nobody ever looked at me as though I were going to die," she recalls gratefully. "They let me know that the way to beat cancer was through *me*. Such care and concern! It made me feel good to be surrounded by people who would back me and help me. All my questions were answered. Even the survival rates were told to me with such positive feelings that I wasn't afraid."

When Nancy's tests were complete, a team of doctors reviewed her case and suggested treatment. The choice was hers: to travel their route, to try simpler treatment, or to eschew treatment entirely.

She chose to go along with the specialists' plan for her— five to six weeks of irradiation from a linear accelerator, followed by two years of chemotherapy, with immunotherapy simultaneous with the chemotherapy.

After ten days in Houston, Nancy returned home for three weeks in order to gain further use of her arm before radiation. For the treatment, it would be necessary to lift her arm and clutch a post, and remain very still.

Beams from the high-powered linear accelerator penetrate deeply, and don't spread to injure healthy tissue. With these advantages over the older cobalt radiation method, it would seem to be the preferred treatment.

The difficulty is that there is a short supply of linear accelerators and of doctors trained to use them. Nancy might have returned to Houston for treatment but fortunately for her, there was a qualified doctor in Dallas, and Nancy's sister lived in Dallas.

Moving in with her sister, going out to lunch daily, suffering not one bit of unpleasant reaction to the five-days-a-week therapy, Nancy claims that she was "Queen of the Hill." So busy was she that she found no time to brood, no time truly to register what had happened to her.

Later, much later, the loss of her breast caught up with her emotionally, and she grieved.

After the Dallas experience, Nancy went home to mother her children and spoil her husband, and to be spoiled in turn. It was an intimate and cherished time.

The couple's strength was bolstered by friends experienced with mastectomy. The women, in essence, said, "Look at me! I made it!" Wanda's husband sought out Nancy's husband, and discussed at length with him the feelings of men in their common situation. Men, indeed, suffer their own unique sadness even as they insist, "It doesn't matter."

Nancy returned to Houston to begin chemotherapy. She was put on a "28-day protocol" with two treatments during each of twenty-eight days, for a period of two years. On "day 1" adriamycin was to be administered intravenously. On "day 8" Nancy was to receive cytoxan (cyclophosphamide) in the form of pills to swallow, and 5-RU (5-fluorouracil) as a liquid to be mixed with orange juice. She also was to participate in a test immunological program.

Adriamycin is a whammy of an anti-tumor antibiotic. Its doses are measured according to the volume of the patient's body, with a lifetime maximum. It must be handled with extreme care. If it escapes the vein, it kills tissue; photographs of such abuse are hideous to view.

Nancy responded normally to initial treatment at M. D. Anderson, and she was cleared to go home. There, her own internist administered the adriamycin in his office, and Nancy was monitored carefully.

In nine months her course of adriamycin ended and

methotrexate was substituted. This was administered by a nurse intramuscularly, by injection into the hip.

Although Nancy suffered a reaction which she describes as head-in-the-jon after every treatment, she never once considered quitting. Her life was at stake, she knew. The adriamycin reaction began late in the day of treatment with "throwing up the pit of my stomach," continued the second day with weakness and backaches, and concluded on the third day with normality seeping back slowly.

There was yet another medical process—BCG—assigned to Nancy.

"It probably will be known as the granddaddy of immunological research. I'm in medical literature!" she says in awe. "All this hopefully will someday lead to a pill that will prevent cancer.

"It is known that cancer depresses the immune system. What BCG does is to introduce a tuberculin bacillus into the patient's system, alerting the body's immune system to fight. When this system is in the habit of fighting, it is hoped it will also battle infections and cancer cells."

How logical. How simple.

But the jury still is out.

For Nancy and her husband, BCG meant a monthly ordeal during which he prepared a two-inch-square area of Nancy's upper arm or upper leg by scratching ten horizontal and ten vertical needle strokes, each stroke deep enough to draw a tiny bit of blood. Into this prepared area a solution was dripped, then dried with cold air from a hair dryer. The area was covered with a plastic lid for twenty-four hours while the solution seeped slowly into Nancy's system, leaving its entry-point red, puffed, and tender. In healing, the spot became crusty and hard.

"My husband did the scratching, and he hated the process more than I did," Nancy remembers. "Eventually, we had to scratch over former sites, and my skin was extremely tender. I still have scars where we accidently cut too deep."

She reports, "The tests aren't conclusive yet, but nobody in my BCG test group had an illness during our two years of testing."

During those two difficult years Nancy ran her household. She maintained a social life. She traveled with two other recent mastectomees across the state to view "a style show for women who have had breast surgery."

All the fashions featured flouncy sleeves, roomy bodices, high necklines. . . . Nancy and her companions giggled through the entire show. They saved their venom for later, in their shared motel room.

Nobody understands mastectomy until she has had one.

In great glee the three women panned the show, lashed out against the public's misunderstandings about breast surgery, expressed anger at secretive doctors. . . .

They shared a beautiful, intimate, laugh-filled evening.

"We ought to have a club!" one announced.

Thus Bosom Buddies was born.

Nancy constantly battles lymphedema, the swelling which occurs when lymphatic vessels or nodes are obstructed or missing. Strains and heavy lifting bring on arm swelling. So do hot, muggy days. Should Nancy iron clothes without wearing her elastic sleeve, she pays the price the next day, spending hours with her arm in the sleeve of a Jobst machine, which she owns. As the sleeve inflates and deflates, it slowly pumps the fluids from Nancy's arm back into parts of her body that remain protected by the lymphatic system.

Would Nancy undergo mastectomy again? And irradiation? And chemotherapy? And BCG?

Yes, with no hesitation at all. Her family needs her.

And she enjoys being alive.

1977

SANDY

"I talk about my experience with anybody who asks," Sandy admits with a pleasant grin. "Maybe this way I can convince women to do regular breast self-examination. Maybe I'll keep somebody from traveling my path.

"I was so dumb about the whole thing! The summer before my surgery I would come into the house from swimming and fix my hair while still wearing my bathing suit. The mirror showed me how fat I was getting, including new fat high on my right breast.

"'I've got to do something about that,' I nagged myself, meaning diet, not a medical ordeal.

"The tumor was enlarging, and I never guessed I had one.

"It is my habit to read sitting up in bed, and as I held a book in front of me, I began to see and wonder about a rippling effect on my right breast. It certainly wasn't a lump, as I expected a lump to be. In fact, I was never able to feel any thickening with my fingers.

"It had been years since I'd been to the doctor—another stupidity of mine. At age forty-seven, I was overdue for a checkup. A little sheepish, I phoned for an appointment.

"No sooner did I mention 'breast irregularity' than I had a same-day appointment."

The rippling was on the upper outer quadrant of Sandy's right breast.

"Doesn't look good," the doctor said, frowning.

Sandy's mammogram was positive, showing a spot the size of a quarter, with "fingers" extending from it.

Having visited an internist and a radiologist, Sandy now consulted a surgeon. All three doctors told her that she probably had cancer.

Three years before, her mother-in-law had died of cancer which had begun in the breast.

Sandy's surgeon wanted to operate immediately. Sandy chose to wait until her husband returned home from a business trip.

"What difference will three more days make?" Sandy argued.

"Probably not a lot," the surgeon agreed.

So they waited.

After two days in the hospital for pre-surgery tests and a bone scan ("staging"), Sandy underwent a mastectomy of her right breast. Her breast and twenty-six of the twenty-eight removed lymph nodes were cancerous.

"They wouldn't tell me how many nodes were involved," Sandy remembers wryly. "They just said, 'Quite a few.' Later, I found out myself by reading my records."

Seven days after surgery, Sandy left the hospital, feeling fine. Ahead of her stretched six weeks of irradiation treatment and then two years of chemotherapy—and she wouldn't feel truly tip-top again until all the treatment ended, until the battle for her life was waged and won.

When Sandy's surgical incision healed sufficiently, cobalt irradiation began. Five days a week, for six weeks, Sandy reported to a radiology clinic.

The first day, a radiologist determined the exact area to be treated, and outlined it with black dye applied with "a sort of magic marker."

"About the time it quits rubbing off on your clothes," Sandy recalls, "they redo the markings."

Sandy's area for treatment included the entire region of her surgery plus a small spot on the back. She remembers the uncertainties of that first day. "You don't know what they're getting ready to do, or how it will affect you," she says.

Shaky with bewilderment, Sandy was taken to a thick-walled room and told to lie on the table. A bulky, sophisticated machine was the room's only other furnishing.

Her body was placed just so; the machine was moved and focused. Warning, "Don't move," the technician left the room.

Sandy didn't move.

The cobalt machine buzzed its prescribed minutes, then went silent.

The technician returned to rearrange Sandy's body, to refocus the machine.

Again the isolation.

Again the buzz.

Not a big deal, Sandy thought with relief.

She was into her third or fourth week of treatment before she developed a lump in her throat. Her voice became raspy, and she coughed.

Later she noticed "sunburn" on the back of her shoulder, reddened skin, where beams of radiation from the cobalt left her body. Although the radiation beam enters the body focused on a specific spot, it spreads as it travels through the body so that its exit area is larger than its entry spot. Upon exiting, it tends to leave the skin reddened.

"These symptoms were nuisances," Sandy admits, "but truly, I never was 'sick' during the six weeks of radiation. Sickness came later, with chemotherapy."

Chemotherapy—the treatment of disease by drugs—was to follow Sandy's cobalt radiation therapy. "Chemo" is handled in our small city, but Sandy opted to go for consultation to the M. D. Anderson Hospital and Tumor Institute in Houston.

"It is my belief that they prescribe stronger drugs there," Sandy says. "Some of them seem to be the last-resort, terminal type medication."

Before Sandy left for Houston, one of her home town doctors told her, "Don't accept anything experimental. Don't be a test case."

"I don't intend to," she assured him.

Even drugs classified as "experimental" have been carefully tested. What is not yet known is the long-term success record of new drugs, or of certain drug combinations. Is the survival rate five years, ten years, fifteen. . . ? Only the passage of time can build statistics.

Chemotherapy is not yet a guaranteed cure.

In Houston, Sandy's case was studied and her "protocol" determined, the protocol being her individual drug prescription. There were to be liquids and pills to swallow, injections into her hip, and medication by the slow intravenous process. Sandy's total time of treatment would be two years.

Sandy's protocol called for three drugs, the two milder ones constant over the two-year period, the powerful adriamycin replaced by methotrexate after the first six months. The administration of adriamycin was stopped a little short of the lifetime maximum dosage, holding some in reserve, should Sandy need it in the future.

"Adriamycin is guaranteed to make you lose your hair," Houston doctors warned Sandy.

They didn't josh. Her hair went fast. Because chemotherapy drugs attack rapidly dividing cells, they hit not only the misbehaving cancer but also the normal fast-growing cells of hair follicles, bone marrow, skin, intestines, stomach, and mouth. This causes the side-effects common (but not inevitable) to chemotherapy patients.

Sandy reached M. D. Anderson Hospital and Tumor Clinic only ten months after Nancy's first consultation there. In the interim, a switch had been made from the twenty-eight-day to a twenty-one-day protocol for breast cancer patients. The drugs were being administered somewhat differently, also.

Sandy underwent her initial treatments in Houston and then returned home. There, on every "Day 1," she reported to the emergency room of a local hospital, where her own internist inserted a tiny needle into a vein in the back of her hand. Drugs administered thus, intravenously, were the powerful adriamycin, mixed (unlike Nancy's protocol) with 5-FU and cytoxan.

Because adriamycin is so tricky to handle, Sandy was monitored closely by the emergency room nurses. It took the major part of a morning for all of the fluid to drip into her veins, time Sandy spent reading or gabbing with medical personnel who dropped by.

On "Day 8," Sandy received a booster of 5-FU and cytoxan, forced rather than dripped into a back-of-the-hand vein. This procedure did not take a lot longer than an injection, and was accomplished in her internist's office.

"Day 21" overlapped "Day 1," and it was back to the hospital emergency room for Sandy.

In common with all other chemotherapy patients, Sandy was given a blood count prior to each of these treatments. Should an abnormal count appear, the scheduled treatment would be postponed. Too-severe reactions would result in cutbacks, too.

The constant watchfulness over Sandy included an EKG every three weeks; potent drugs can damage the heart. Kidneys, too, are at risk.

When adriamycin was removed from Sandy's protocol after six months, the intravenous sessions ended. Then she received methotrexate in the hip, cytoxan in the form of pills to swallow, and 5-FU as a liquid which she mixed with water and drank.

Chemotherapy made Sandy ill, a flu-type illness complete with weakness, headaches, body aches, and vomiting. Soon, she learned to block after-treatment days from her calendar; they were lost days, as far as accomplishment or socializing were concerned.

Sandy blames her broken arm on weakness from therapy. She fell. Fortunately the break did not occur on the side of her mastectomy, which would have complicated healing, because of the lost lymph nodes and vessels.

As the break healed, Sandy asked her doctor, "What can I do to regain the use of my arm?"

He growled, "You already know what to do to regain the use of an arm, don't you?" Sandy had been diligent in exercising, and her mastectomy-affected arm functioned adequately.

"Near the end of the two years, I was sick of being sick," Sandy recalls. "To this day I can't look a Certs breath mint in the face because those blue specks on Certs are just like the blue specks on the cytoxan I swallowed, and then promptly vomited. Toward the end, I was vomiting all medication. No drug seemed to stay down."

Now, comfortably beyond chemotherapy, Sandy looks back with humor. In her view, treatment with drugs had certain advantages over and above its main goal of keeping her alive. Didn't menstruation cease with her very first treatment? Isn't her new growth of hair glossier and thicker than before? Wasn't she temporarily freed from the chore of shaving legs and armpits? Wasn't her face amusing with eyebrows and eyelashes missing?

Nowadays Sandy refuses to be introspective. "There isn't any point in delving into feelings," she claims. "Cancer is here. A reality. We cope when it's necessary to cope."

Being in a higher risk category, because breast cancer seems to be at least in part hereditary, Sandy's daughters have learned to self-examine. "They'll never be blind, as I was, to changes in their breasts. They'll never ignore annual checkups, as I did," Sandy hopes.

"My family was wonderful, she praises. "They supported my chemotherapy treatment although they knew I was entering into a long period of sickness. Really, I wasn't worth anything for two entire years."

Family and friends remember differently. They remember an unchanged Sandy, going forward at full speed.

Except, that is, for a few days following each treatment.

1979

ESTHER

Troubles in her past had squeezed Esther emotionally, and from time to time she sought help from a psychiatrist. She spoke frankly of her mental history, confident that she had "got it all together." Smooth sailing seemed to stretch ahead.

Then at age fifty, she underwent a modified radical mastectomy. There was no lymph involvement, no post-surgery treatment.

"I'm going to make it," she marveled. "This isn't going to get to me." She continued an active social life.

The third month after surgery, she became introspective. The reality of cancer haunted her more and more.

The fourth month she dropped her long-favorite activities as well as her newer ones: Bosom Buddies and Encore. She also became a dropout from all contact with her friends, and they could do nothing except worry because she rejected all overtures.

Wisely, she returned to psychiatric treatment, enlisting professional help to tide her over a period of despair. Now she is a smiling and social creature once again.

1980

IRIS

"I didn't think there was anything unusual in the way I came through mastectomy," Iris confides. "I was out of the hospital three days after surgery. In ten days I flew to Dallas to visit friends, and we shopped all the time. I had no therapy or treatment of any kind, and I've had no trouble since."

Iris was sixty-seven years old when, in 1980, a close friend underwent mastectomy. Alerted by this, Iris checked her own breasts and to her dismay discovered an oddity the size of a nickle. Within days it elongated, reaching toward the nipple.

Her mammogram was negative, yet her doctor urged biopsy.

Iris entered the hospital, prepared to acknowledge cancer and to expect mastectomy, an attitude which her surgeon recommended.

"I thought: it could be cancer, and if it is, it is." Iris shrugs, remembering.

When she awoke from anesthetic she explored her bandages with her fingertips and knew her breast was gone. Her bosom had been ample, so there was no doubt.

That night a nurse entered Iris's room and demanded sharply, "What are you doing?"

"I'm on my way to the bathroom," Iris answered reasonably.

"You're not supposed to be up," the nurse scolded.

The weakness that Iris felt during this premature walk was the only weakness that she ever has experienced. By the next morning she was strolling the hospital halls. In three days she returned home to ordinary housewifely chores, suffering no post-surgery fatigue.

Iris's mastectomy had been a modified radical, with

eighteen—but not all—of the lymph nodes removed. The nodes tested negative. Iris's cancer had been caught early, because her friend led the way.

That friend is a focus of Iris's concern. Her cancer had spread. She accepted cobalt treatment but refused chemotherapy.

"So far, she's doing fine," Iris reports, her worry for her friend unconcealed.

Iris recalls that until about 1970 she was unaware of mastectomy among her acquaintances. Were fewer women having breast surgery? Or were they not talking?

One of the non-talkers, when finally confronted, told Iris, "Well, I think if I don't talk about it, it'll go away."

Iris's personal rebellion is in the form of a refusal to submit to mammograms of her remaining breast. She has lost faith in mammography.

She also suspects that she would not again rush into surgery. Instead, she would explore the alternative treatments that have received so much airing in the press. Only after she was equipped with up-to-date survival rates would she decide for, or against, another mastectomy.

CONCLUSION TO CASE HISTORIES

Fourteen women.

Fourteen humans with little in common except breast surgery.

Never do they feel victimized.

Or tragic.

Certainly not handicapped.

Theirs is not a veneer of bravery, easily cracked. Perhaps personal strength is a byproduct of mastectomy.

Fourteen women. What do their stories tell us?

In almost every case, discovery of a lump or thickening was made, quite by accident, by a woman who did not regularly practice breast self-examination.

The lumps and thickenings differed, one from another. Some grew with terrifying speed, some barely changed. Some were biopsied upon discovery, others were watched for months or years.

A common medical decision seems to be to wait and watch.

Is it wise? Judging from my case and others, I think not. It might be possible to wait and watch all the way to the cemetery. I feel strongly that suspicious breast lumps should be biopsied and examined.

Physicians are in a difficult position, of course. They are accused of ordering too many expensive tests, too many exploratory surgeries. The estimate that nine out of ten biopsied breast lumps are benign may support their wait and watch position. Also, there is some risk involved in any surgery, even a biopsy.

Oddly, the strongly hereditary pattern of breast cancer

did not show up in this small study. Of these fourteen women, only Nancy had a relative with breast cancer.

The twelve who were married at the time of mastectomy emphasized the roles of their husbands in bolstering their self-esteem. They continued to be sexy, desirable creatures; their husbands made that clear. Not one woman hid to undress or wore a concealing brassiere and prosthesis to bed. Sex life did not change except perhaps for the better, cancer being a reminder that each partner is mortal.

If a husband over-reacts to breast loss, his wife will, too.

All of the interviewed women expressed a common complaint: that their surgeons did not provide sufficient information to prepare them for possible physical and mental after-effects of mastectomy. About one-third complained that medical personnel "treated us as though we didn't have a brain in our heads."

Often these women failed to elicit answers because they didn't know how to phrase questions. Their reading on the subject was catch-as-catch-can; and consequently, they are ardent supporters of the relatively new Reach to Recovery program, with its informative and instructional pamphlets as well as its personal I-too-walked-this-path approach.

When doctors did dictate certain post-mastectomy rules, their restrictions led to confusion. Gloria was bowling with her right arm within six weeks of her right-breasted radical surgery, yet none of us is to carry suitcases or even purses in our mastectomy-affected arms because of possible strain. We must remain active, yet careful. How our instructions collide!

As I interviewed the thirteen living mastectomees, I kept prodding for their fears. Do they see themselves as alive and well in five years, ten years, twenty. . . ?

Indeed they do.

Perhaps I am the most fearful of all, although my fear is not of cancer, but rather of a too-early end to life.

By no means do I intend to suggest that the cancer centers named in these case histories are superior to others elsewhere. They just happen to be ones that are frequented by people in the southwestern United States. Fine facilities and compassionate staffs are our true blessing, wherever we live.

Cancer treatment rides on shifting sands. Not long ago, it was virtually routine to follow mastectomy with radiation. Now, radiation is used more selectively. New drugs are introduced, medications are combined in new ways, old faithful potions and procedures fall into disuse. Records of every success and every failure contribute toward the day when cancer may be conquered.

Never pity a mastectomee. Instead, rejoice with her that her disease was discovered in time to wage war against it.

Fourteen women. One dead at age ninety-three, thirteen very much alive.

Women with little in common except breast surgery.

Never do they feel victimized.

Or tragic.

Certainly not handicapped.

They harbor no grudges; they rush out to meet life full force. They squeeze joy from each day.

And they thank God for each day, knowing that He was merciful.

GLOSSARY

Adenoma   A tumor of glandular origin and structure that usually is benign or of low-grade malignancy.

Adriamycin   An antibiotic which is toxic to tumor cells.

Adrenalectomy   The surgical removal of two small endocrine glands, one above each kidney, which supply ten per cent of the body's estrogens.

Aspiration   Removal of fluid or tissue by means of a hypodermic syringe.

Autoclave   To sterilize by superheated steam in a pressure vessel.

Axilla   The armpit, the location of axillary lymph nodes.

BCG   An immunological research project.

Benign tumor   An abnormal swelling or growth that is not a cancer and is usually harmless.

Bilateral   On both sides.

Biopsy   The surgical removal of tissue from a living subject for microscopic examination in order to make a diagnosis.

Bone scan   A method for detecting bone cancer. A chemical which is attracted to bone is "tagged" with a radioactive element and injected into a vein. The chemical behaves differently in a cancerous tumor than in normal cells. A radiation detector is moved over the entire body several hours after the injection to measure concentrations of the radioactive element in various bones.

Breast self-examination (BSE)   Procedure by which a woman checks herself once a month for cancer symptoms.

Cancer   A large group of diseases characterized by uncontrolled growth and spread of abnormal cells.

Carcinogin   Any substance that causes cancer.

Carcinoma in Situ   A stage in the growth of cancer when it is still confined to the tissue in which it started.

Chemotherapy   Treatment of disease by chemical compounds.

Cyclops   1. Any of the three one-eyed Titans who forged thunderbolts for Zeus in Greek Mythology. 2. Any of a race of one-eyed giants, reputedly descended from these Titans, inhabiting the island of Sicily.

Cyst   An abnormal sac that is firm, smooth, and round, and that contains a liquid or semi-solid material that can be aspirated. It is tender on palpation or pressure, and usually is harmless.

Cytoxan (Cyclophosphamide)   A chemical used in chemotherapy. It is an alkylating agent which arrests cell division.

EKG (Electrocardiograph)   An instrument used to record electric currents through the heart for the purpose of detecting abnormal heart functions.

Encore   The YWCA Postmastectomy Group Rehabilitation Program.

Endometriosis   The spilling of cells which normally line the uterus.

Estrogen   A hormone secreted by the ovaries and adrenal glands.

Estrogen-binding study (Estrogen-receptor assay)   A test to determine to what extent a cancer is stimulated in its growth and reproduction by the presence of estrogens.

Fibrosis   The formation of ropelike tissue in excess of amounts normally present.

Fibrocystic breast disorder   The condition in which fibrous tissue obstructs a woman's mammary ducts so that trapped fluids swell the ducts to form cysts. These benign cysts enlarge and deflate with the menstrual cycle, unlike cancerous lumps which remain the same or grow. Additional terms for this condition include fibrocystic breast disease, sclerosing adenosis, ductal dysplasia, mastasia, and chronic cystic mastitis.

5-FU (5-fluorouracil)   A chemical used in chemotherapy. It is an antimetabolite which destroys cells by depriving them of their needed vitamin folic acid.

Halstead radical mastectomy   Removed are the breast, the lymph nodes in the axilla, and the pectoral (chest) muscles.

Hemovac   A vacuum device for draining a wound. (Fluid builds up under the skin after tissue is removed, and must be drained away.)

Hormones   Chemical substances that help to regulate growth, metabolism and reproduction.

Immunotherapy   Treatment of disease by stimulating the body's own defense mechanism against the disease.

Irradiation   Same as radiation therapy.

Keloid   An overgrowth of scar tissue.

Linear accelerator   A straight tube maintained under vacuum

through which atomic particles are accelerated to high speed
and thus high energy.

Lumpectomy   Surgical removal of a cancer and only a small amount
of its surrounding tissue.

Lymph   A clear, watery, albuminous fluid which circulates
throughout the body, containing white blood cells, antibodies
and nourishment to clean, protect and feed body tissues.

Lymphedema   Swelling which occurs when lymphatic vessels and/
or lymph nodes are missing or obstructed.

Lymph nodes   Oval-shaped filters located along the vessels of the
lymphatic system to clean debris (such as worn out cells) and
microorganisms (including infection-laden bacteria and cancer cells) from the lymph fluid. Unfortunately the nodes
sometimes nourish the trapped cancer cells.

Malignant tumor   A tumor made up of cancer cells that grow and
invade surrounding tissues and sometimes break away to
grow elsewhere.

Mammogram   X ray of the breast for diagnosis of cancer.

Mastectomee   A woman who has undergone mastectomy.

Mastectomy   Surgical removal of a breast, especially of a cancerous breast to prevent spread of the disease.

Metastasis   The process by which cancer cells break away from the
original tumor and start new malignant tumors elsewhere in
the body; the malignant spread of a cancer to another organ.

Methotrexate (MX, Amethopterin)   Another chemical used in
chemotherapy which functions as an antimetabolite.

Modified radical mastectomy   Removal of the breast and axillary
lymph nodes, retaining the chest muscles.

Oncologist   A doctor who specialized in the study and treatment of
cancer.

Oophorectomy   The surgical removal of one or both ovaries to halt
the ovaries' production of cancer-feeding hormones.

Palpation   Examination with the hands.

Pathologist   A doctor who examines the tissue and fluids of a body
to learn the nature of disease, its causes, processes, development and consequences.

Pectoral muscles   The chest muscles.

Prosthesis   An artificial replacement for a missing body part. Plural:
prostheses.

Protocol   Standardized procedures followed by doctors so that the
results of treatment may be compared.

Radiation therapy   Directing high energy radiation (X rays, gamma rays, or the like) into cancer cells in order to kill the cells.

Radiologist   A doctor who specializes in using radiant energy in the diagnosis and treatment of disease.

Reconstruction   The implanting of a silicone breast form in the chest of a mastectomy patient.

Recurrence   Appearance of a second cancer in the general area of the first.

Sclerosis   A thickening or hardening of a body part especially from tissue overgrowth or disease.

Serum hepatitus   Inflammation of the liver caused by a transfusion of contaminated blood.

Simple mastectomy (Also called total mastectomy)   The breast is removed; the lymph nodes and chest muscles are retained.

Staging   Finding the extent of the cancer's growth and spread so as to determine its most effective treatment.

Tumor   An abnormal mass which performs no useful body function. It can be cancerous or benign.

Unicorn   A fabled creature usually represented as a horse with a single spiraled horn projecting from its forehead and often with a goat's beard and a lion's tail.

X ray (Noun)   Radiation similar to light, but of an extremely short wave length. These rays have the ability to penetrate solid bodies. They are used in medicine for both diagnosis and treatment.

X-ray (Verb, Adjective)   To irradiate with X rays.